CONSULTING TO CHAOS

FORENSIC PSYCHOTHERAPY MONOGRAPH SERIES

Series Editor: Professor Brett Kahr
Honorary Consultant: Dr Estela V. Welldon

Other titles in the Series

Violence: A Public Health Menace and a Public Health Approach
Edited by Sandra L. Bloom

Life Within Hidden Worlds: Psychotherapy in Prisons
Edited by Jessica Williams Saunders

Forensic Psychotherapy and Psychopathology: Winnicottian Perspectives
Edited by Brett Kahr

Dangerous Patients: A Psychodynamic Approach to Risk Assessment and Management
Edited by Ronald Doctor

Anxiety at 35,000 Feet: An Introduction to Clinical Aerospace Psychology
Robert Bor

The Mind of the Paedophile: Psychoanalytic Perspectives
Edited by Charles W. Socarides

Violent Adolescents: Understanding the Destructive Impulse
Lynn Greenwood

Violence in Children: Understanding and Helping Those Who Harm
Edited by Rosemary Campher

Murder: A Psychotherapeutic Investigation
Edited by Ronald Doctor

Psychic Assaults and Frightened Clinicians: Countertransference in Forensic Settings
Edited by John Gordon and Gabriel Kirtchuk

Forensic Aspects of Dissociative Identity Disorder
Edited by Adah Sachs and Graeme Galton

Playing with Dynamite: A Personal Approach to the Psychoanalytic Understanding of Perversions, Violence, and Criminality
Estela V. Welldon

The Internal World of the Juvenile Sex Offender: Through a Glass Darkly then Face to Face
Timothy Keogh

Disabling Perversions: Forensic Psychotherapy with People with Intellectual Disabilities
Alan Corbett

Sexual Abuse and the Sexual Offender: Common Man or Monster?
Barry Maletzky

Psychotherapy with Male Survivors of Sexual Abuse: The Invisible Men
Alan Corbett

CONSULTING TO CHAOS
An Approach to Patient-Centred Reflective Practice

Edited by
John Gordon and Gabriel Kirtchuk
with
Maggie McAlister and David Reiss

Routledge
Taylor & Francis Group
LONDON AND NEW YORK

Excerpt from *Happy Moscow* by Andrey Platonov, translated by Robert & Elizabeth Chandler. Published by The Harvill Press and reproduced by permission of The Random House Group Ltd.

First published 2017 by
Karnac Books Ltd.

Published 2019 by Routledge
2 Park Square, Milton Park, Abingdon, Oxon OX14 4RN
52 Vanderbilt Avenue, New York, NY 10017

First issued in hardback 2019

Routledge is an imprint of the Taylor & Francis Group, an informa business

British Library Cataloguing in Publication Data

A C.I.P. for this book is available from the British Library

ISBN 13: 978-0-367-10266-1 (hbk)
ISBN 13: 978-1-78220-126-7 (pbk)

Typeset by Medlar Publishing Solutions Pvt Ltd, India

We dedicate this book to the memory of Professor Gill McGauley who died after a brief illness before she was able to see the proofs of her chapter, Attachment, Mentalization and the Interpersonal Dynamics Consultation. Gill's outstanding theoretical, clinical, and organisational contributions to the field of forensic psychotherapy are greatly appreciated by her colleagues and friends

CONTENTS

ACKNOWLEDGEMENTS

We are very grateful to the service managers and professional colleagues who over many years have supported the development of the Interpersonal Dynamics consultation and participated so honestly in the multidisciplinary consultations themselves. Those involved in the weekly Interpersonal Dynamics consultation workshop, including Richard Ingram and colleagues in Belfast, Moustafa Saoud and colleagues in Chichester and others throughout the UK, have made a major contribution to refining our understanding of the ID framework and the role of the ID consultant in a variety of settings.

A big thank you to Alexander (Aggie) Ashman for generously offering one of his many phantastic paintings for our cover!

The Introduction contains material regarding the history and administration of the Interpersonal Dynamics consultation previously published by the editors of this volume as *Interpersonal Dynamics Consultation: A Manual for Clinicians*, London: Imperial College and West London Mental Health NHS Trust, 2013.

The epigraph to the Introduction is from *Happy Moscow* by Andrey Platonov, translated by Robert & Elizabeth Chandler. It is published by The Harvill Press and reproduced by permission of The Random House Group Ltd.

The research project described in Chapter One was originally carried out for a doctoral dissertation awarded in 2011 by the University of Essex.

An earlier version of Chapter Eight appeared in *Psychoanalytic Psychotherapy* 30: 182–195, 2016, and we thank the editor of that journal for permission to use it in a different context here.

We especially appreciate Rod Tweedy, Kate Pearce, Kate Morris and Cecily Blench at Karnac for their patient and expert shepherding through the process of publication.

And, last but never least, to Brett Kahr, the Forensic Psychotherapy Monograph Series Editor, who enthusiastically encouraged us from the start: Muchísimas gracias otra vez.

ABOUT THE EDITORS AND CONTRIBUTORS

Richard Church is a Consultant Psychiatrist and Lead Clinician at Lambeth CAMHS, South London and Maudsley NHS Foundation Trust, and an Honorary Clinical Senior Lecturer at the Institute of Psychiatry, Psychology and Neuroscience, King's College London. He has a background in child and adolescent psychiatry, and forensic psychiatry, with a particular interest in the mental health of young people in conflict with the law. He serves on the executive committees of the Adolescent Forensic Psychiatry Special Interest Group (AFPSIG) at the Royal College of Psychiatrists, and the European Association for Forensic Child and Adolescent Psychiatry, Psychology and other involved Professions (EFCAP).

Ronald Doctor is a Consultant Psychiatrist in psychotherapy and forensic psychotherapy in the West London Mental Health NHS Trust and a member of the British Psychoanalytical Society. He has had a number of roles in postgraduate and undergraduate medical education including Training Programme Director, West London Higher Training Scheme in medical psychotherapy and forensic psychotherapy, and Site Coordinator for undergraduate medical training, Imperial College, London. He was Chair of a number of national organisations among them the Association for Psychoanalytical Psychotherapy in the NHS and the NHS Liaison Committee, British Psychoanalytical Society. He is the Regional Representative, London Division, and was the Academic Secretary, Psychotherapy Faculty, at the Royal College of Psychiatry. He has edited two books, *Dangerous Patients: a psychodynamic approach to risk assessment and management* (2003) and *Murder: a psychotherapeutic investigation* (2008). His most recent peer publication is "History, murder and the fear of death" in the *International Journal of Applied Psychoanalytic Studies*, 2015.

Dr. Amber Fossey is a 2006 medical graduate from University College London and registered Psychiatrist with a Bachelor's degree in psychology and a Masters in psychotherapeutic approaches in mental health. She is currently specialising in forensic psychiatry at West London Mental Health NHS Trust and working at Broadmoor High Secure Hospital.

John Gordon is a Full Member of the British Psychoanalytic Association and Senior Member of both the British Psychotherapy Foundation and the Institute of Group Analysis. Previously he was Consultant Adult Psychotherapist in a forensic psychotherapy department and at the Cassel Hospital. He is Senior Lecturer at Buckinghamshire New University where, in collaboration with West London Mental Health NHS Trust, he co-organises, teaches, and facilitates an experiential group on an MSc in psychodynamic approaches in mental health. He is co-author with the late Stuart Whiteley of *Group Approaches in Psychiatry* (1979), co-editor of *Psychic Assaults and Frightened Clinicians* (2008), and co-author of *Interpersonal Dynamics Consultation: A Manual for Clinicians* (2013). He has published many papers on the development of Bion's thinking on psychosis and its application to clinical work with individuals, groups, and organisations. He currently practices privately as a psychoanalyst and supervisor.

Dr. Richard Ingram is a Consultant Psychiatrist and psychoanalyst who works full time in the Belfast Health and Social Care Trust. He provides medical psychotherapy services to regional forensic and general psychotherapy services. He also has a keen interest in psychoanalytic training and is Chair of the Northern Ireland Association for the Study of Psychoanalysis, a member institution of the British Psychoanalytic Council.

Professor Gabriel Kirtchuk is a Consultant Psychiatrist in Psychotherapy (Forensic) and a Fellow of the British Psychoanalytical Society. He is the Head of the Forensic Psychotherapy Department at West London Mental Health NHS Trust where, in collaboration with Buckinghamshire New University, he developed and is co-leader of an MSc in psychotherapeutic approaches in mental health. Over the years he and his colleagues have developed a manual which facilitates the systematic study of transference/countertransference patterns by means of consultations with multidisciplinary teams, particularly in in-patient forensic settings; more recently this approach has been extended to services in the community as well as generic psychiatric, child, and adolescent settings. Until recently he was Lead Clinician of the National Forensic Psychotherapy Training and Development Strategy, a post he held for many years. He is an Honorary Senior Lecturer at Imperial College Medical School and Chair of the Forensic Psychotherapy Society, a Member Institution of the British Psychoanalytic Council (BPC).

Julian Lousada is a psychoanalyst with the British Psychoanalytic Association, past Clinical Director of the Adult Department at the Tavistock & Portman NHS Trust, and past Chair of the British Psychoanalytic Council. He now works in private clinical and organisational practice.

Jose Maret is a Dual Training Specialist Registrar in medical psychotherapy at the Ealing Forensic Psychotherapy Services at St Bernard's Hospital. He has a special interest in group analysis and is doing his Masters in psychotherapeutic approaches in mental health with Buckinghamshire New University. He is currently involved in setting up an Interpersonal Dynamics (ID) consultation service for the non-forensic psychiatric local services in the area.

Colin R. Martin, RN, BSc, MSc, PhD, MBA, YCAP, FHEA, C.Psychol, AFBPsS, C.Sci, is Professor of Mental Health at Buckinghamshire New University, Middlesex, UK. He is a Registered Nurse, a Chartered Health Psychologist, and a Chartered Scientist. He also trained in analytical biochemistry, this aspect reflecting the psychobiological focus of much of his research within mental health. He has published or has in press well over 200 research papers and book chapters. He has written and/or edited fifteen books, all of which reflect his diverse academic interests that examine in-depth the interface between mental health and physical health. These include the *Handbook of Behavior, Food and Nutrition* (2011), *Nanomedicine and the Nervous System* (2012), *Comprehensive Guide to Autism* (2014), and *Diet and Nutrition in Dementia and Cognitive Decline* (2015). Professor Martin promotes strongly an interdisciplinary approach to clinical research, evidence-base development, and innovative scholarly activity. Examples include his book, *Comprehensive Guide to Post-Traumatic Stress Disorder* (2016), a multi-volume treatise covering this distressing clinical presentation. Additionally, he has major research programmes focusing on stress-vulnerability models of psychosis and schizophrenia, perinatal mental health, puerperal psychosis, occupational wellbeing assessment, forensic psychiatry, addiction, myalgic encephalomyelitis, and, as highlighted, the relationship between physical and mental health. He is involved in collaborative International research with colleagues in many countries.

Maggie McAlister is a Jungian Analyst with the Society of Analytical Psychology and works as a Principal Adult Psychotherapist in a forensic psychotherapy department in a medium secure unit within the NHS. She originally worked as a Dramatherapist in adult mental health settings and has written and published extensively on her work as an Arts Psychotherapist and Adult Analyst in forensic and adult psychiatry. She is a registered supervisor and senior lecturer for the MSc in psychotherapeutic approaches to mental health jointly run by West London Mental Health Trust and Buckinghamshire New University. She has a private practice in North London.

Professor Gill McGauley MBBS, MD(Res), FRCPsych was Professor of Forensic Psychotherapy and Medical Education at St George's University of London and a Consultant in Forensic Psychotherapy in Central and North West London Foundation NHS Trust (CNWL). In CNWL she developed and delivered psychotherapy services for women in HMP & YOI Holloway and HMP & YOI Bronzefield. She previously worked at Broadmoor where she established the first Forensic Psychotherapy service in a high secure hospital. She has developed national and international training and educational initiatives in forensic psychotherapy as Chair of the National Reference Group for Training and Education in Forensic Psychotherapy and through her work for the International Association for Forensic Psychotherapy. At St George's she was Head of The Centre for Clinical Education. Her research focused on the application of attachment theory and the development of psychological therapies such as Mentalization Based Treatment (MBT) for personality disordered offender patients. She was awarded a National Teaching Fellowship by the Higher Education Academy in recognition of individual excellence in teaching in the UK.

Aikaterini Papaspirou recently completed the Higher Specialist Training in Forensic Psychotherapy at the Portman Clinic scheme: she trained at the Tavistock and Portman NHS Foundation Trust and at the West London Mental Health NHS Trust. She is currently working as a Consultant in forensic psychiatry in West London. She has published a book review on *The Murderess*, a novella by Alexandros Papadiamantis, in the *Journal of Forensic Psychiatry and Psychology*. She has also contributed a chapter in *Forensic Group Psychotherapy: The Portman Clinic Approach* (2014), published by Karnac.

David Reiss MA, MBBChir, MPhil, PgD, FRCPsych, FAcadMEd is a Consultant Forensic Psychiatrist for West London Mental Health NHS Trust and Honorary Clinical Senior Lecturer at Imperial College London. His research interests are in the interface between clinical forensic psychiatry and public policy, including work on personality disorder, recidivism, homicide inquiries, and educational issues. His clinical and educational work focuses on enabling the multidisciplinary team to gain an enhanced understanding of patients, thereby improving care and reducing risk. He is co-editor of *Containment in the Community: Supportive Frameworks for Thinking about Anti-Social Behaviour and Mental Health* (2011) and co-author of *Interpersonal Dynamics Consultation: A Manual for Clinicians* (2013).

Beate Schumacher is a Fellow of the British Psychoanalytical Society and works as an Adult Psychotherapist in the NHS in a forensic psychotherapy department as well as in a Tier 2 outpatient psychotherapy service; previously she worked for many years at the Cassel Hospital's Family Service. She is a Senior Lecturer for the MSc in psychotherapeutic approaches in mental health run jointly by West London Mental Health Trust and Buckinghamshire New University. In addition to her NHS work, she maintains a private practice, teaching, and supervising both in the UK and abroad.

Dr. Maja Turcan is a Consultant Clinical Psychologist currently working in private practice and in the third sector, prior to which she worked for more than twenty years in the NHS, specialising in forensic and secure services. She has worked extensively with patients with complex disorders and histories of abuse and trauma. Her work has included staff support and supervision. Whilst working in the NHS she was involved in management and service development, focusing on new approaches to working with women in secure services. Currently, in addition to clinical work she is working with adult survivors of childhood abuse and trauma, and with staff who work with Holocaust survivors.

SERIES EDITOR'S FOREWORD

As every practising mental health professional will know only too well, working with patients can be a very taxing experience. Not only do we spend much of our days listening to tales of trauma and misery, but at times, our more distressed patients will enact their historical furies upon *us*. Indeed, they may insult us, scream at us, or even institute proceedings against us—an increasingly common occurrence in our litigious world—often for no good reason other than the fact that we have the capacity to bear such outbursts and even encourage such outbursts in true psychoanalytical spirit.

No wonder, then, that even Sigmund Freud, the progenitor of the "talking cure", often found his clinical activities taxing and enervating and, at times, infuriating. For instance, in a moment of tremendous frankness, Freud (1918a, p. 142) wrote to his cherished Hungarian colleague, Dr Sándor Ferenczi, that, "Nicht alle Fälle, die ich jetzt habe, sind auch interessant. Manche sind einfach quälerisch" ["Not all the cases that I have now are also interesting. Some are simply agonizing"] (Freud, 1918b, p. 273).

Freud could, however, be even more blunt. One decade later, he wrote to another Hungarian physician, Dr István Hollós, about his hatred of psychotic men and women: "Ich gestand mir endlich, es komme daher, dass ich diese Kranken nicht liebe, dass ich mich über sie ärgere, sie so fern von mir und allem Menschlichen empfinde" (Freud, 1928a) ["Finally I confessed to myself that I do not like these sick people, that I am angry at them to feel them so far from me and all that is human"] (Freud, 1928b, p. 537).

An uncharitable mental health practitioner might regard Freud's seemingly cruel comment as an indication that he had embarked upon the wrong career and that he should have remained a neurologist ... or should even have become, perhaps, a lawyer or an accountant!

But the British psychoanalyst Dr Donald Winnicott would have understood Freud's hatred completely. In 1947, Winnicott presented a landmark paper entitled "Some Observations on Hate" to his colleagues at the British Psycho-Analytical Society, published two years later, in 1949, under the title "Hate in the Counter-Transference", in which he underscored that treating psychotic patients places a tremendous burden upon the clinician, and that it would not be at all unusual for a psychoanalyst to experience an "*Objective Hate*" (Winnicott, 1949, p. 72) towards his or her patients.

Freud and Winnicott wrote from the perspective of being solo practitioners, working in private practice settings, with one patient at a time. But what happens when the mental health specialist must deal with many ill patients simultaneously, on the ward of a psychiatric hospital, or in a secure forensic unit, or in some other communal setting? How does the practitioner bear or tolerate the multiple stresses and projections that devolve from undertaking such work with so many highly traumatised and traumatising individuals?

Treating highly complex patients within an institutional setting demands a great deal of internal fortitude and, also, a tremendous amount of collegial support. But in the absence of such ideal conditions, workers often find themselves becoming depressed or acting out aspects of the patients' psychopathology.

I shall never forget one of my old teachers at the Portman Clinic from decades ago, who had consulted extensively to a variety of mental health institutions. This gentleman told me how frequently his colleagues, when treating genital exhibitionists, would leave case files lying about—*exposed*, in fact—so that anyone could read the patients' notes. Likewise, he recalled that colleagues who worked with paedophiles would often engage in ugly arguments during staff meetings, in which one member of the team would end up feeling infantilised and then abused, as if raped by an older person. These forensic dynamics percolate and then penetrate all too viscerally and all too frequently.

Back in 2008, John Gordon and Gabriel Kirtchuk, two highly experienced London-based psychoanalysts and forensic specialists, published a volume in our "Forensic Psychotherapy Monograph Series", memorably entitled *Psychic Assaults and Frightened Clinicians: Countertransference in Forensic Settings* (Gordon & Kirtchuk, 2008), in which they and their fellow contributors, all accomplished psychoanalytical workers, explored the impact of dangerous patients, housed in institutions, upon those who endeavour to help them. This lucid and helpful book immediately outstripped all other titles in our forensic monograph series in terms of sales—no doubt an indication that many colleagues found themselves struggling with the problem of how to survive "burnout" and "compassion fatigue" in such challenging settings.

It pleases me greatly that nearly one decade later, Gordon and Kirtchuk have produced a follow-on text, *Consulting to Chaos: An Approach to Patient-Centred Reflective Practice*, edited in association with fellow forensic colleagues Maggie McAlister and David Reiss (the latter a contributor to the earlier book (Kirtchuk, Reiss, & Gordon, 2008)). I can happily describe this new book as well worth the wait.

In a series of deftly argued chapters, written by a team of highly accomplished professionals from the interrelated fields of forensic psychiatry, forensic psychotherapy, clinical psychology, group analysis, psychoanalysis, and Jungian analysis, the authors explore how mental health clinicians endeavour to cope with chaos in the consulting room and, moreover, on the ward or in the institution more broadly. The essays draw upon classical psychoanalytical theory (and, in particular, the works of Melanie Klein and Wilfred Bion) and, also, upon more contemporary conceptualisations, which include attachment theory and mentalization.

This book will be of immediate assistance to front-line workers in all branches of the mental health professions and will have useful implications for those in other public sectors, not least among physicians and nurses and social services specialists too. The concept of "Interpersonal Dynamics" explored in this volume will, I predict, have immediate reverberations among many grateful people keen to fortify their working situations.

The chapters speak for themselves, and I shall not, therefore, provide a summary. But I do wish to celebrate that the publication of this particular book—the seventeenth title in our "Forensic Psychotherapy Monograph Series"—provides strong evidence of just how impactful the field of forensic psychotherapy has become in recent years. When we launched our series back in 2001, only one colleague, to the best of my knowledge, held a formal post in forensic psychotherapy in the British National Health Service, but now, more than fifteen years later, quite a number enjoy such positions, not least the majority of contributors to this book.

Nowadays, Great Britain boasts not only a training in forensic psychodynamic psychotherapy, established many years ago by Dr Estela Welldon, but also a Forensic Psychotherapy Society, as well as many departments of forensic psychotherapy within the public sector, which sit alongside the pioneering International Association for Forensic Psychotherapy. Additionally, we have two monograph series in this country devoted to the subject. Furthermore, the Royal College of Psychiatrists sponsors a Forensic Psychotherapy Special Interest Group. Indeed, Professor Gabriel Kirtchuk, the co-editor of this volume, holds the position as Lead Clinician of the National Forensic Psychotherapy Training and Development Strategy. And shortly before her untimely death in 2016, our much-loved and much-missed colleague, the late Dr Gill McGauley—a contributor to this book—became the country's first Professor of Forensic Psychotherapy and Medical Education at St George's Hospital Medical School in the University of London. The discipline has even spawned offspring in the shape of forensic art psychotherapy, forensic disability psychotherapy, forensic mental health nursing, forensic music psychotherapy, and other branches. "Forensic psychotherapy" even has its own Wikipedia page!

I congratulate the editors for having assembled such a fertile and creative team of leading contributors, whose work not only provides helpful insights into the management of the chaos of organisations but also offers concrete evidence that psychological thought has at last penetrated to the depths of the institutions which house some of nation's most dangerous citizens.

Professor Brett Kahr
Series Editor
Forensic Psychotherapy Monograph Series
London

References

Freud, S. (1918a). Letter to Sándor Ferenczi. 17th March. In: Sigmund Freud and Sándor Ferenczi (1996). *Briefwechsel: Band II/2: 1917–1919*. Ernst Falzeder, Eva Brabant, Patrizia Giampieri-Deutsch, and André Haynal (Eds.), pp. 141–142. Vienna: Böhlau Verlag/Böhlau Verlag Gesellschaft.

Freud, S. (1918b). Letter to Sándor Ferenczi. 17th March. In: Sigmund Freud and Sándor Ferenczi (1996). *The Correspondence of Sigmund Freud and Sándor Ferenczi: Volume 2, 1914–1919*. Ernst Falzeder, Eva Brabant, Patrizia Giampieri-Deutsch, and André Haynal (Eds.). Peter T. Hoffer (Transl.), pp. 272–273. Cambridge, Massachusetts: Belknap Press of Harvard University Press.

Freud, S. (1928). Letter to István Hollós. 10th April. Box 15. Freud Museum, Swiss Cottage, London.

Freud, S. (1928). Letter to István Hollós. 10th April. Peter Gay (Transl.). Cited in Peter Gay (1988). *Freud: A Life for Our Time*. New York: W.W. Norton.

Gordon, J., & Kirtchuk, G. (Eds.). (2008). *Psychic Assaults and Frightened Clinicians: Countertransference in Forensic Settings*. London: Karnac.

Kirtchuk, G., Reiss, D., & Gordon, J. (2008). Interpersonal Dynamics in the Everyday Practice of a Forensic Unit. In John Gordon and Gabriel Kirtchuk (Eds.) *Psychic Assaults and Frightened Clinicians: Countertransference in Forensic Settings* (pp. 97–112). London: Karnac.

Winnicott, D. W. (1949). Hate in the Counter-Transference. *International Journal of Psycho-Analysis, 30*: 69–74.

FOREWORD

by Julian Lousada

Reading this book leaves me feeling two things: first, pride in the creativity of psychoanalytic application and, second, anger that the case for a reflective practice has to be made over and over again. This book demonstrates a remarkable commitment to understanding very disturbed patients in their in-patient and community settings—patients who alarm themselves and frighten others. It argues that understanding how the patient impacts on the professional might represent the most valuable way of understanding what is going on in the patient's mind, especially for those patients who cannot, or dare not, understand themselves. The book's proposition is "that exploring interpersonal aspects of a patient's early and later relationships, in addition to an inspection of events preceding violence, can greatly enhance the deduction of triggers to violence and improve risk assessment" (p. 81), as well as contributing to an understanding of interactional dynamics and vicious cycles that impede effective treatment.

The authors have developed an application of Interpersonal Dynamics (ID) such that consultation within rehabilitative units and amongst multidisciplinary teams can serve to promote early warning signs of violence/risk and unify therapeutic approaches. The development of the ID protocol is very interesting, not least because of its "simple" three way relational focus: a focus on the patient's experience of self and others, a focus on the interpersonal relations and the differing experience of the multidisciplinary team, and a focus on the mind within the systemic context. Out of the interrogation of what is contained in these sites of focus comes the possibility of a better understanding of patients and their therapeutic needs.

Implicitly, the book draws our attention to a correlation between the mental health of the professional team and the quality of the intervention they are able to provide. It highlights the extent to which disturbance in the patient can and does become projected into and identified with by the staff and by the system that provide their care. Such disturbance is not polite or well mannered but raw and in need of containment and understanding. It is in effect a communication from the patient to the system in the hope that there is the capacity to think and process its meaning. Simply put, this book describes a method of organisational consultation that seeks to transform the enactments that flow from being fearful of, angry with, or despairing about the patient into attending to and thinking about the patient.

Furthermore, the book makes an eloquent case for the need for a reflective instrument, which in this case is the ID consultation. It is well researched and theoretically grounded in psychoanalytic ideas. What makes me angry is that we cannot take for granted that a reflective space is understood to be an essential part of a clinical service if the needs of both patients and staff are properly to be kept in mind. My fear is that the thinking in this book, like those it follows, for example Michael Balint, Isabel Menzies Lyth, Elliot Jaques, and Robert Hinshlewood to name but a few, will continue to be seen as a luxury rather than an essential element in the delivery of good practice.

Parity of esteem between physical and psychiatric care can only be taken seriously if and when it is understood that the fear of contact with serious mental disturbance has to be overcome. Parity, if it means anything, implies an ambition for change. Change in the context of mental distress is seldom triumphant and frequently modest, but whatever is possible is a product of an engagement and the relationships that this suggests.

INTRODUCTION

The Interpersonal Dynamics (ID) consultation: context, rationale, history, and method

John Gordon and Gabriel Kirtchuk

> The spherical hall of the restaurant, deafened by the music and the howls of people, and filled by the tormenting smoke of cigarettes and the gas of squeezed passions, seemed to revolve; every voice in it sounded twice, and suffering kept on being repeated. It was impossible here for anyone to break free from the ordinary—from the round ball of his head, where his thoughts rolled on along tracks laid down long ago, from the bag of the heart, where old feelings thrashed about as if they had been netted, accepting nothing new and letting go of nothing to which they were accustomed—and brief oblivion in music, or in love for a woman one had happened upon, ended either in irritation or in tears of despair. The later time got and the more the merriment thickened, the quicker the restaurant's spherical hall began to revolve; forgetting where the door was, many of the guests span around in terror on the spot, somewhere in the middle of the hall, supposing they were dancing. (Platonov, 1999/2001, pp. 83–84)

Introduction

This book is about how to survive and to develop the capacity for creative work in organisations and community settings where professionals and severely ill patients encounter one another. These organisations and settings have been called "toxic institutions" (Campling, Davies, & Farquharson, 2004) in which participants are "irradiated by distress" (Hinshelwood & Skogstad, 2002) as they "suffer insanity" (Hinshelwood, 2004) and worse—utter terror—particularly in confronting the simultaneously murderous and decimated minds of the forensic patients with which many of the following chapters are concerned. In *Psychic Assaults and Frightened Clinicians: Countertransference in Forensic Settings* (Gordon & Kirtchuk, 2008), we characterised the experiences of staff members as akin to those of Creon in Seneca's visceral version of *Oedipus*: "I saw every torment every injury every horror spinning like flames and shadows/sickening forms faces mouths reaching up clutching/towards us and crying" (Hughes, 1969, p. 34). The invasive, "clutching" quality of experience in the extreme clinical settings described by the authors of this book underscores the importance of a conceptual framework which can function as a mental seat belt for staff by giving meaning to what would otherwise lead to drowning in dread, reacting in rage and/or escaping through a kind of professional distancing (Hinshelwood, 1999) which can only be sustained by ruthless attacks on perception, feeling, and thinking: murdering one's own experience in a bizarre, tragic identification with the murderous patients. For us this underlying framework is psychoanalytic, specifically an understanding of the transference–countertransference dynamics between individuals (patients and various members of multidisciplinary staff teams involved in their care and treatment) as well as within and between the multiple (sub)groups which comprise the organisation.

Essentially, we have adapted features of Kleinian psychoanalytic thinking and its development by Bion to understand transference–countertransference dynamics at individual, group, and organisational levels. First, the intense polarisation of emotional experience in the paranoid-schizoid mode is fundamental to understanding clinical work with severely ill patients. Loving and hating become radically intensified—total and totally separated—as do the loved and hated figures: idealisation or destruction reigns in an omnipotent, infinite, timeless "now". Destruction in particular has been acted out repeatedly and often devastatingly by this patient group.

Second, projective identification is the fundamental means by which these patients clutch the feelings, minds, and very personalities of those who work with them. Projective identification (Bion, 1962/1984, 1967/1984, 1970/1984; Joseph, 1989; Klein, 1946, 1955; Meltzer, 1992; Money-Kyrle, 1956; Ogden, 1982; Pick, 1985; Rosenfeld, 1987; Segal, 1986; Sodre, 2015; Spillius, 1988a, 1988b; Spillius & O'Shaughnessy, 2011; Steiner, 1993) consists of (1) an omnipotent, unconscious evacuative phantasy that it is possible to sever (split off) from the personality any function (perception, thinking, feeling) or content (specific feelings, thoughts or memories)—whether negatively or positively evaluated—which arouses intolerable anxiety or pain and to deposit it into another person; and often (2) a real interpersonal impact which induces the recipient(s) to experience something like the evacuated aspects of the projector. It is a desperate defence of a beleaguered mind which can operate at one extreme to enhance phantasies of control over others and to eliminate any sense of separation or difference in order to deny dependence: in effect, there may be no "patients" who acknowledge a need for care in the settings described in this book (Gordon, 2004). This psychic surgery and transplant operation infuses every aspect of the organisation and its members. On the other hand, projective identification is a potential and fundamental means of communication; for if the recipient(s) of projective identifications can attend to their emotional experiences and thoughts they might garner clues to the ways in which the projector has contributed to the interaction and to the motives involved.

Finally, following from the preceding point, the concept of containment (Bion, 1959, 1962, 1970) or mentalization (Bateman & Fonagy, 2004) of the transplanted/evoked mental functions and contents by the recipient(s) is a *sine qua non* of effective individual and coherent multidisciplinary team intervention. Containing involves recognising, staying with and thinking about the possible sources and meanings of evoked feelings. Consequently, countertransference becomes a crucial focus of clinical work (Gordon & Kirtchuk, 2008). The terrifying revolutions of the dance to oblivion described by Platonov is an apt metaphor for the inevitable failures to contain the ubiquitous enactments and dramatisations of attacks on others and on the patients' own minds ("lack of insight", "negative symptoms") which characterise clinical work on the edge (Gordon, Harding, Miller, & Xenitides, 2005). Furthermore, it describes the constant recycling of projective identifications as staff members in turn dump the intolerable states evacuated into them into colleagues, members of other professions, other wards or departments, managers or, dangerously escalating the pace of the dance, back into a particular patient or into the patient group.

Our focus in this book, the Interpersonal Dynamics (ID) consultation as a method of facilitating patient-centred reflective practice, is a central component of what we referred to as a mental seat belt for staff, a means to find a space from which reflection on the whirling "gas of squeezed passions" might be possible and within which a process of recognising, acknowledging, evaluating, and organising the elements and patterns of this toxic gas can occur in order to alter the interpersonal context of the secure treatment environment. Accordingly, the ID consultation is an experiment in applied psychoanalytic thinking. We will further elucidate some of the psychoanalytic underpinnings of the ID consultation below.

Context: reflective practice

More generally, a reflective space (Gordon, 1994; Hinshelwood, 1994) in the form of weekly reflective practice (or work-study) groups for staff is acknowledged as an essential, frequently advocated if far from consistently available aspect of clinical work in mental health settings. Its necessity arises from the nature of severe mental illness and personality disorder as well as from the task complexity for a multidisciplinary group to organise multiple treatment interventions into a coherent whole, all the while adapting these interventions to the idiosyncratic regressions/developments of individual patients over time.

The patients described in this book, who are characteristic of those met with in a variety of hospital, prison and community settings, to a greater or lesser extent are unable to handle their perceptions and feelings in the usual way. They can feel as bombarded by their sense perceptions, emotions, and imaginings as though by a material event like a tsunami. One extremely violent patient said, "Anger happens." His feeling was a brutal assault, not the subjective response of an interpreting self. And typically, via the projective phantasy that it is possible to separate that lump of rage from his personality, he would get rid of the persecuting stuff within by immediately inflicting it on others who would be left helpless, damaged, and enraged. Samuel Beckett describes a related phenomenon in *Malone Dies* (1956) during an interaction between Lemuel, a psychotic patient, and MacMann, his nurse:

> But Lemuel was made of sterner stuff, in this connection, and far from being a stickler for the statutes seemed to have little or no acquaintance with them. Indeed the question might have arisen, in the mind of one looking down upon the scene, as to whether he had all his wits about him. For when not rooted to the spot in a daze he was to be seen, with heavy, furious reeling tread, stamping up and down for hours on end, gesticulating and ejaculating unintelligible words. Flayed alive by memory, his mind crawling with cobras, not daring to dream or think and powerless not to, his cries were of two kinds, those having no other cause than moral anguish and those, similar in every respect, by means of which he hoped to forestall same. Physical pain, on the contrary, seemed to help him greatly. And one day rolling up the leg of his trousers, he showed Macmann his shin covered with bruises, scars and abrasions. Then producing smartly a hammer from an inner pocket he dealt himself, right in the middle of his ancient wounds, so violent a blow that he fell down backwards, or perhaps I should say forwards. But the part he struck most readily, with his hammer, was the head, and that is understandable, for it too is a bony part, and sensitive, and difficult to miss, and the seat of all the shit and misery, so you can rain blows upon it, with more pleasure than on the leg for example, which never did you any harm, it's only human. (Beckett, 1956, pp. 267–268)

Such patients are also often convinced that what they see, feel and think is equivalent to a camera taking perfectly accurate pictures of the world. They believe their thoughts and feelings about situations and other people are the only possible way to understand them. Finally, they often don't take into account before acting the perspectives of the other people around them who may have been involved in the interactions which prompted their feelings in the first place. Instead thoughts and feelings, as in the quotation above, are more like stuff clogging up their bodies and heads and causing intolerable tensions. This almost physical experience makes hanging on to their reactions long enough to really know them and think about them just about impossible. Consequently, with forensic and other patients with complex conditions, action discharge replaces reflective function often in the form of breaking boundaries. Hammers, or their emotional equivalents in the form of projective identifications, are often directed at staff members' heads and personalities.

This chronic deficit in patients' reflective capacity ("lack of insight" or "amnesia" regarding the index offence, as Treasaden describes (2003)), as well as the resulting tendency to act rather than to think, are naturally expressed in the treatment setting as in all other areas of the patients' lives, past and present. This might sound weird, but imagine it in the following manner: on the ward and in the hospital patients empty their minds through patterns of relating to and communicating with staff. Patients can't or don't want to know what is going on in their own minds and in their lives, which have frequently been traumatic for themselves and for others. So instead they can behave and talk in certain ways and so manage to stir up in other people something like the feelings and thoughts and experiences that they are rarely able to grasp or actively seek to avoid. Sometimes just reading a patient's case history or suddenly hearing from a family member what a patient has done to get admitted to a secure hospital might be enough to have a devastating effect on anyone. This doesn't even begin to take account of patients' undermining, intrusive, or threatening behaviour on the ward. Therefore, communicating and relating under the conditions of reflective deficit and the action mode are often through emotional (and sometimes physical) impact on individual members of staff and on the staff team as a whole.

In the treatment setting, patients' problems in thinking and their tendency instead to act meet up—and not infrequently clash—with staff's provision of care, treatment, and security. This makes for a complicated and sometimes confusing mix. Carrying out a professional role vitally depends on staff finding creative methods to bring together care, treatment, and security in *response—not re-action*—to engagement with patients. The problem is that when patients make their impacts on staff the ordinary result can be a human reaction, usually an emotional reaction which may not lead to an action but will certainly be felt strongly by the staff. Sometimes it is very difficult not to react to the patient's stimulating impact with a counter-action. Many of these emotional impacts are painful, difficult, or bewildering. And staff members' emotional reactions also sometimes seem to contradict what a good professional is "supposed to feel" toward patients. Nevertheless, whatever goes on in a staff member's mind while relating to a patient might represent a most valuable understanding of what is going on in the patient's mind, especially if it is a patient who doesn't want to or can't understand herself. Some patients may communicate and relate similarly with all members of the multidisciplinary team (MDT), while others may have very contradictory effects on different staff. It is only by combining these varied impressions that an in-depth, realistic view of the patient may be reached. As individuals and as members of MDTs, professionals need a regular opportunity to stand back and think about the turbulent interactions and impacts which make up everyday life on the wards.

The unique purpose of a Reflective Practice Group is to offer this regular opportunity for staff members to reflect together on their work as individuals and as a team. In particular, by sharing openly their experiences of working with patients and with one another—both positive and negative—professionals may be able slowly to restore the meanings lost to patients whose minds can no longer consistently make sense but who may give others clues as to what is going on for them. On the basis of possible new understanding arising from reflection on their own responses, staff will be in a better position as individuals to avoid playing into patients' maladaptive agendas and as a team to make their multiple interventions more coherent and comprehensible to patients. Sometimes they may also be able to feed back their understanding to the patients and to see how they respond.

Accordingly, reflective practice is potentially most useful and effective

- When it is at a time when as many staff as possible can attend
- When all professions within the MDT are represented
- When there is an agreement regarding confidentiality
- And when each participant is supported to talk about his work experiences as openly and honestly as possible, as well as to listen respectfully to others' honest and frank responses.

However challenging, when these conditions are met it is possible over time to build up a meaningful account of patient-staff interactions in an extremely difficult and complex work setting for the benefit of both patients and professionals. Here is an example of what can happen in an "ordinary" reflective practice group.

I (JG) came onto the secure ward of a forensic hospital where several weeks previously I had arranged to meet regularly with multidisciplinary professionals to discuss their work. We had agreed the time and place, but on the first two occasions I had found myself alone for fifteen minutes. When I went out of the appointed room to ask at the nursing station whether people were planning to come to our reflective practice, I was informed that it hadn't been put in the diary for that week. Eventually my appearance outside the glassed-in nursing office would be noted, and members of the staff would file into our room.

Shortly after this inauspicious "launch" of the group, I was sitting with the consultant psychiatrist, a nurse, and a health care assistant. The consultant, a regular attendee and major force behind the initiation of the group, was wondering aloud to his nurse colleagues whether any more of their peers intended to come. They were at a loss, commented that the ward was "very busy today" and we all lapsed into a perplexed, helpless silence tinged with annoyance at what was pretty clearly emerging as resistance to, if not outright sabotage of, the reflective practice. I was not particularly surprised by this reluctance which I had experienced many times in forensic and other staff groups—including ones to which I belonged as a participant rather than a facilitator. But I had never experienced what was about to happen in this reflective practice group.

Suddenly the door opened and six male staff members burst into the room. Their faces showed utter perplexity while we were startled and stared as they stood, silently towering over us for what seemed forever. Finally I asked what was going on. To our collective amazement, one of the arrivals managed to stammer that they had just been called by the nurse in charge—this ward was divided into two geographically separate areas, one acute, the other a smaller rehabilitation section where they had been telephoned by the charge nurse on the acute ward where the group takes place to respond to an emergency. The spokesman, increasingly joined by his incredulous co-responders, told us that, arriving on the ward, they had been directed by the nurse in charge to the reflective practice room where they were expecting to find a dangerous, aroused patient causing chaos and possibly severe damage to their colleagues. They could not believe their eyes to find four people sitting in silence around a table, and we could not believe what we were being told.

Eventually, the "response team" joined us at the table; we continued for a while to grin at each other trying to absorb the implications of what we had just witnessed; and then some of these implications began to be spelled out, both in this meeting and others that followed. For reflective practice had suddenly been energised by our joint experience. The members of the "response team" expressed their sense of having been utterly betrayed and lied to by a senior colleague. How could they have been set-up in such a serious and frightening way by members of their own profession? This sentiment was seconded in spades by those who had already been in the meeting. Amazement gave way to anger and then to a despairing cynicism which reconfirmed for many that no one could be trusted in such a dangerous setting. But this event seemed to show that even members of your own professional tribe would not be watching your back. On the contrary, they might deliver you into the hands of the enemy.

Many succeeding reflective practice meetings were spent in trying to identify this dangerous enemy as .... thinking about their work at all. Whether it was a deceptive senior colleague, a manager, or I myself who might be held responsible for forcing them to attend reflective practice; even an unconscious and disowned part of one's own mind advocating the usefulness and survival value of thinking creatively under pressure to "make the best of a bad job" (Bion, 1979), this object could not be perceived as authoritative, helpful, and caring but only as treacherous, attacking, and destabilising. Through dramatising the latter quality, we began to understand how the charge nurse had reflected this negative internal presence, patently corrupt, unworthy of loyalty and respect and mandating fight/flight. At a subsequent meeting we found out more about the anxieties which maintained such an ominously malevolent image of authority.

I arrived to find a number of group members already present, passing around and laughing over a brochure on the table. The main theme of the meeting was that managers only came to the ward to criticise, otherwise you never saw them. And if a patient complained about you, the investigation would be arduous: a third degree. Examples from group members' experiences were given. As I was listening I found myself trying to decipher the, for me, upside down writing on the cover of the brochure, which had ended up at the other end of the table from where I was sitting. It dawned on me that this was an advertisement for a theme park roller coaster, and the name of the ride emerged: NEMESIS INFERNO!!! I said that I thought this was exactly what they feared reflective practice was; and that by demonising it—helped immeasurably by the nurse in charge whose deception had legitimised their (and his) continuing rebellion against attending—it was possible to protect themselves as a team from anxiety that open engagement in the group could only reveal humiliating individual inadequacy, failure, and probably worse qualities in themselves. They believed that contacting their feelings about the work would contaminate their ability to continue to care for their patients.

We are still riding the roller coaster. But that is what working in secure forensic settings is. The proto-constituents of the "minds" of forensic patients, including inchoate and unmetabolised emotional states, are externalised and dispersed though their interactions with staff on the ward, just like the real damage they have already wreaked in the external world. And among the emotions which some patients may never be able to tolerate, and others become psychotically depressed or acutely suicidal when they approach, is persecuting guilt: a constituent of the NEMESIS INFERNO which turned up in our reflective practice group.

The ID consultation: rationale

The ID consultation (Kirtchuk, Gordon, McAlister, & Reiss, 2013) is a highly structured method of group reflective practice. It provides a clear protocol (see Appendix I at the end of the book for the worksheet and cluster/item list which form the basis of the ID consultation) which enables all staff who know the patient—from senior manager to consultant psychiatrist to ward cleaner—to discuss their interactions. Everyone knows in advance that a specific patient has been referred to a consultant, trained to meet with the widest possible range of professionals/agencies involved in that patient's care, management, and treatment, in order to describe and discuss the relationship patterns enacted between the patient and significant past and present figures, including the staff who are currently most acutely involved. Since the task of group participants is explicit and focussed, many of the intense, destabilising anxieties triggered by group membership itself (Bion, 1961; Gordon, 2011), which can threaten the very survival of the group as illustrated in the above example, are alleviated sufficiently to allow participants to proceed with their task.

In clinical work, an awareness of patients' subjective experiences, particularly their perceptions of interpersonal relationships, is indispensable. The aim of this book is to improve care and treatment planning by describing and supporting a methodical approach to eliciting patients' core relationship patterns. These patterns consist of the roles and scenarios into which they repeatedly cast themselves and others with whom they interact. Maladaptive patterns, in which vicious cycles and self-fulfilling prophecies of misperception, misunderstanding or provocation escalate, cause pain and havoc in personal relationships and can adversely affect both professionals' decisions and the overall delivery of treatment. We are concerned to show how to use vital information that is often not made available to treatment teams in order to understand such potential pitfalls rather than succumb to them.

Routine clinical meetings in mental health settings, such as ward rounds, usually involve discussion of patients' symptoms and behaviour. This focus, which derives from the *Diagnostic and Statistical Manual of Mental Disorders 5* (APA, 2013) and the *International Classification of Diseases* 10 (WHO, 1994) frameworks, is essential. However, it does not include the wealth of untapped information embedded in the complex and often subtle interpersonal communications arising from the working relationships between patients and staff. Our premise is that formalised psychiatric evaluation and risk management are immeasurably enhanced by systematic exploration of these interpersonal scenarios as they emerge in the treatment context.

Modern mental health services are essentially multidisciplinary and multi-agency. The team approach to caring for and treating patients, based on shared goals, competencies, and capabilities, is a central clinical and political imperative. Nevertheless, often opposing this objective is the reality that different professions organise their interventions separately and employ different languages with limited conceptual and clinical overlap, sometimes to the detriment of patient care.

Beyond the effects of continual changes regarding professional roles and identities imposed by professional and governmental policies, there are two additional factors that contribute to a lack of working together in institutional and community care—often with the kinds of catastrophic consequences attributed by formal inquiries to systemic failures of communication: the interpersonal context, and the organisational context. In the first of these, the professions tend to go in different directions as a result of pressures arising from the interpersonal impact of patients' dysfunctional behaviour and communication. There is an active process by which individual members of multidisciplinary teams and agencies, as well as the separate professional groups themselves, are differentially perceived, used, valued, and devalued by patients. When members of one profession, say nurses, feel devalued by patients, compared to doctors who are idealised, it becomes more difficult for the two disciplines to cooperate together.

Patients who have suffered from abuse or neglect in early childhood and perhaps also experienced victimisation as adults may, without realising what they are doing, influence others through the repetition of previous adverse interpersonal patterns. People with these difficulties are found in all areas of psychiatric and social work and are especially prominent in forensic settings. Usually we can recognise them by the strong emotions they are able to generate in staff. For example, some are able to divide the team's views on how they should be managed. Others may elicit intensely positive or negative feelings in specific members of staff. In the extreme, an outsider listening to the various strands of a team case discussion might think that different team members were describing two completely separate patients.

The second factor which can lead to less than optimally coherent service delivery is based on a psychodynamic/systems theory of organisations (Armstrong & Rustin, 2014; Hinshelwood & Chiesa, 2002; Hinshelwood & Skogstad, 2000; Hirschhorn, 1995; Jaques, 1955; Menzies Lyth, 1960). All members of staff must struggle to create a picture in their minds of the overall objectives of their organisation and to be aware of how their roles link with each other in order to fit in with these objectives. The work that they have been set up and authorised to do, not by themselves alone but by multiple stakeholders in the organisation's external environment, cannot be accomplished if staff do not have a game plan and the resolve to stick to it. Failure to achieve the objectives—whether converting raw materials into cars for sale or transforming minds acutely disturbed on admission into more stable mental states prepared for discharge—means failure of the organisation.

To stand any chance of completing the job by means of integrating their roles, members of an organisation must be in touch with the reality of the work, but in many mental health settings, this reality is extraordinarily painful and frightening. To survive and navigate their everyday encounters with a work reality infused with the fragmented minds of patients, expressed through impact in dysfunctional interpersonal scenarios, individual members of staff deploy their own resources to cope with the aroused anxieties, emotions, and impulses. Such individual self-protective strategies are based on the life experiences and personalities of each organisational member and are, consequently, more or less mature. However, organisations, like all groups, "offer" their members shared or group-level methods of protection to bolster their individualised attempts to shield themselves from the destabilising emotional glare of direct contact with patients. These shared procedures are group norms, generalised prescriptions on how to carry out the work which may be taught formally, as part of explicit organisational training procedures, or are informally, often implicitly, absorbed as individuals are initiated into the organisation's ways of doing things. Jaques (1955) and Menzies Lyth (1960) referred to such group/institutional-level processes as "social defences".

Like individual coping strategies, the group-sanctioned methods of operation may be more or less mature: more or less in touch with the reality of the work. Unless they are conceptualised and subjected to evaluation, such normative working routines, while they may enable staff to survive and remain in their settings, characteristically pull the direction of their energies and efforts away from the primary aims of the organisation. A central finding of research based on this organisational perspective is that the normal, adaptive division of functional roles becomes splintered and fragmented: organisational functioning comes to mirror and reiterate the very disordered states it is meant to transform. Different professional groups may start to concentrate on partial, and therefore "manageable", aspects of the work; they may even focus exclusively on different aspects of the patient in isolation from the particular focus of other colleagues. Anxiety intrinsic to the reality of facing an integrated task evaporates in the reassuring refrain that patients are "settled", while managers complain that nurses remained in their offices throughout the shift and nurses complain that doctors and therapists are only on the ward for a limited time. Blame is passed around, along with feelings of inadequacy. Paradoxically, some familiar, almost automatic and "settled", working practices may increase the possibility of organisational failure, a completely unintended consequence of an understandable and necessary quest for security.

To overcome all of these inescapable centrifugal forces, we believe it is vital for each clinical team to develop an explicit framework to organise its clinical practice so that gaps in communication can be monitored and addressed. Specifically, the different professionals involved in a patient's care must meet regularly to coordinate their separate views based on certain shared concepts and a common language. By doing this all staff, even if they come from different theoretical backgrounds, can work in partnership to interpret and understand the observed behaviour and symptoms of the patients, as well as their responses to the various treatment interventions.

The consultation described in this book is a further development of the Operationalised Psychodynamic Diagnostics (OPD), a comprehensive clinical assessment approach which has been described by the OPD Task Force (2001, 2008), Stasch, Cierpka, Hillenbrand, and Schmal (2002), Stasch (2004), Dahlbender, Rudolf, and OPD Task Force (2006) and von der Tann et al. (2007). It is able to reveal the underlying dynamics of a patient's interactions in a way that can be comprehended and contributed to by all multidisciplinary team members. Objectivity, which is seen as the gold standard of scientific measurement, is prized and promoted in contemporary clinical practice, whereas subjective experience, which has traditionally been viewed as not meeting the criterion of detachment, has consequently been marginalised in many forms of psychiatric and psychological discourse. We propose that subjective experience, in particular the ways that staff react to patients and *vice versa*, can be codified, organised, and contextualised so as to make it a valid and reliable tool in routine clinical work.

Interpersonal dynamics

Stable, predominantly positive interpersonal relationships are central to mature personality development and good mental health: they form the matrix of the mind. Unrewarding, painful or hostile relationships are inevitable and, within the context of positive interactions, are not only made safe but contribute to resilience. We usually experience our everyday interactions as a dynamic balance between initiating contacts with others, responding to their approaches, and realising that we and they are also always considering possible interpretations of each other's initiatives and responses which, according to whether they are positive or negative, feed into the relationship and drive it along. To "mentalize" (Bateman and Fonagy, 2004) relationships is to consider simultaneously our own states of mind—motives, wishes, intentions, fears, perceptions, initiatives, and responses—and those of others with whom we are interacting. This contributes to tolerance, to an awareness of uncertainty and complexity, and to an appreciation of nuance and surprise in human relationships.

Our encounters in the clinical setting, however, are often of a different nature and show particular maladaptive characteristics. First, many of our patients have a *limited range* of ways of relating to others. For example, they may tend to see themselves as only needy and dependent and view others primarily as (adequate or inadequate) caretakers. Second, such relationships tend to be employed *repetitively, rigidly, and inappropriately* in a broad range of interactions with others. From a psychodynamic perspective, such inflexible patterns of interpersonal interaction, which may originate in childhood and continue to determine the basic shape of adult functioning, are called transference relationships. A third characteristic of dysfunctional interpersonal interactions is that the patient tends to see himself as merely and perpetually *responding* to the active behaviours of others and pays relatively little attention to how his own approach or impact might affect them. Finally, many of our patients tend to *resort to action* as a response to the perceived motives and behaviour of others, rather than to reflect and try to understand the possible meanings of the interaction. In turn, patients' tendency to act out repeatedly can also impair staff's capacity to think and can lead to counteractions (a form of countertransference) which may include breaking professional boundaries.

In essence, our patients focus actively on their perceptions and interpretations of the manner in which they believe others treat them, as well as reactively responding, primarily by actions and impacts. They are accordingly less able to be aware of their own initiatives and of how these might be interpreted by others. They also do not experience what we have referred to as their active perceptions and interpretations as such; for them these are facts about the other, not products of their own minds which may or may not accurately take account of the reality of others' intentions and behaviour. At its extreme, perceptions and interpretations of self and others' behaviour may take the form of delusional belief. Thus, perception of, interpretation of and influence on current interpersonal interactions are profoundly shaped by unconscious transference repetitions (Gosling, 1968).

Transference and countertransference

We have alluded to the *transference* as a rigid, compulsory repetition in the present of a relationship pattern which originates in the past, typically in infancy and childhood, and which out of awareness continues to habitually inform and be imposed on current interactions with significant figures in the patient's environment. The *countertransference* refers to the counter-responses of the recipients toward whom the patient's transference(s) are directed. Staff (other) countertransference as responsiveness to the patient includes the whole gamut of human emotional, cognitive, and action potential. So patients may "select" from this available pool just the responses which are required to fit their internal scenarios and produce dramatic re-enactments with current others: projective identification is ubiquitous. Of course others are also primed by their own transference patterns, as well as by the understandable effects on them of their patients' impacts, to respond either in accordance with patients' transferences or to resist. In this way, transference–countertransference can be seen as "schemas", the lifelong accumulation of relationship experience in the form of internal working models or cognitive affective schemata (Bowlby, 1973; Horowitz, 1991).

Transference–countertransference configurations enacted between each patient and those members of the staff involved in his treatment often evoke a complementary self relating to other (Racker, 1968) response. For example, the patient plays the role of self, say an appreciative little boy, with one member of staff who responds in the role of a satisfied mother. With another member of staff, the patient in the role of an angry child transfers an attitude of hostile rejection; and the professional feels like a useless mother. With yet a third, the patient repeats the self role (experience) of feeling bad and guilty, while the other is induced to be a critical, rejecting mother.

Roles can be—and often are—reversed when the patient plays the part of "(m)other" while staff are put in the position of the patient's self within the particular transferred scene. It can be very difficult for staff to be cast by the patient in more "negative" roles, for example, when the patient is really pushing us to respond critically or making us feel completely worthless and useless. But it is even harder when the patient, in reversing the roles, succeeds in making us experience what it was like to be her as a child. This can be exceedingly painful, may feel cruel, and can lead to staff attempts to evade the experience. On the other hand, exploring the countertransference offers an exceptional opportunity to get to know the patient from the inside and can enable alternative responses that are less maladaptive and more concordant with the real treatment needs of the patient.

Importance of Interpersonal Dynamics (ID) for clinicians

It is possible, within a multidisciplinary team (MDT) setting, through systematic examination of the information available about an individual patient, to delineate the patterns of dysfunctional interpersonal interactions starting in childhood and continuing in the staff-patient interactions on the ward. Identifying the dysfunctional interpersonal interactions may inform risk assessment and allows the staff to devise specific care plans to help modify the dysfunctional interactions.

Through experience, we know that various members of the MDT highlight differing aspects of the patient which may not be known to colleagues. This sharing of multiple pictures of a patient's personality and behaviour as expressed in their relationships adds to the coherent understanding of the patient by the staff.

A discussion of the staff-patient interactions can, therefore, improve communication within the staff group through provision of a common understanding of the dysfunctional interactions and lead to a more consistent response to patients' behaviour. It can also identify situations in which staff may perhaps have acted out in response to patients' behaviour and enhance the ability of staff to think and reflect. This is turn would reduce the risk that staff would breach professional boundaries.

The ID consultation: historical background

Birtchnell (1993) described how relating, an activity which is universal across the animal kingdom, confers advantages upon those who are successfully able to engage in it. He outlined how relationships could be described by two axes: proximity (horizontal) and power (vertical). Freud (1933) had previously proposed that there were two types of human instinct: sexual and destructive, which corresponded to the horizontal axis, and power relationships, represented by the vertical axis.

Freud's work was taken forward by Sullivan (1953), a psychiatrist and psychoanalyst, who understood that infants need emotional contact with others and that early perceptions of interpersonal interactions, initially with parents, greatly influences adult personality development. His theory recognised that everyone fundamentally requires love and power in order to be secure and free from anxiety. He also emphasised how important it is for mental health professionals to be able to understand the world as the patient sees it.

The "object relations" school of psychoanalytic theory further developed this strand of work and highlighted the paramount importance of attachment (Bowlby, 1969) and autonomy for normal development (Greenberg & Mitchell, 1983).

Bowlby's original concept has been substantially developed by those working in the attachment field to produce a comprehensive and in-depth understanding of attachment behaviours and difficulties in interpersonal relationships. Recent developments in neuroscience (Schore, 2001) have explored how brain and personality development are impaired in infants who experience psychological neglect from primary caregivers. Bateman and Fonagy (2004) have conceptualised this impairment as a deficit in the capacity to mentalize: to represent mental states. The mentalization based approach is highly relevant to interpersonal dynamics as the aim is to increase the capacity for reflective function in order to better understand the emotions, intentions, and beliefs of others, and to differentiate these from those of oneself.

Murray (1938) produced a list of human needs which he saw as themes underlying human behaviour. Leary (1957) conducted empirical research and arranged a selection of Murray's needs around two perpendicular axes (love/hate and dominate/submit) to form the basis of the interpersonal circle. This arrangement, which describes a spectrum of possible interactions that can occur within a relationship, is also known as a circumplex (Guttman, 1996). Schaefer (1965) proposed a vertical axis, modelled on parenting behaviours, which is defined in terms of allowing autonomy versus control.

Allport (1937: 48) defined personality as "the dynamic organisation within the individual of those psychophysical systems that determine his unique adjustment to his environment", and he used the term "dynamics" to refer to an individual's goals and purposes. Benjamin (1996), drawing on both personality theory and the interpersonal circle, produced the Structural Analysis of Social Behaviour (SASB) model. She wanted to develop a more objective understanding of psychopathology in interpersonal terms and demonstrated distinctive relationship profiles for different types of personality disorder. In the forensic context, Blackburn (1998) has used the interpersonal circle to examine the relationship between interpersonal style and criminality in both mentally ill offenders and those with personality disorder. He found that offenders with extensive criminal careers have a more dominant and coercive interpersonal style.

Development of the ID four-perspective consultation

The Operationalised Psychodynamic Diagnostics (OPD) Task Force (2001, 2008; Cierpka et al., 2007; Gross, Stasch, Schmal, Hillenbrand, & Cierpka, 2007; Stasch, Cierpka, Hillenbrand, & Schmal, 2002; Stasch, 2004) have formulated a reliable empirical method to determine stable but dysfunctional patterns in relationships. It took up the circumplex model, was heavily influenced by the SASB (Benjamin, 1996) and elaborated this approach by taking into account the work of others who have also outlined rigorous methods of observing interpersonal interactions (Hoffman & Gill, 1988; Horowitz, 1991; Luborsky & Crits-Christoph, 1990; Strupp & Binder, 1984; Weiss & Sampson, 1986). The totality of OPD is a comprehensive, validated, structured assessment protocol which combines descriptive phenomenological diagnostics (APA, 2013; WHO, 1994) with psychodynamic features derived from psychoanalysis (for reliability and validity data see Cierpka et al., 2007). Patients are assessed on five axes: (I) experiences of illness and prerequisites for treatment; (II) interpersonal relations; (III) conflicts; (IV) structure; and (V) mental and psychosomatic disorders.

In our work with the multidisciplinary team, we concentrate on the framework of Axis II, which concerns the patterns of relationship that characteristically describe patient-staff interactions. Our basic procedure is to conceptualise (adapted from OPD) four perspectives of the patient's core relationship patterns by clarifying (1) how the patient characteristically perceives the other; (2) how the patient responsively experiences himself; (3) how others (including staff members) usually perceive the patient; and (4) how others/staff experience themselves in their interactions with the patient.

The four interpersonal perspectives:

Perspective A: The <u>patient</u> repeatedly perceives <u>others</u> so that they are … (focus is on the other—active)
Perspective B: The <u>patient</u> regularly experiences <u>himself/herself</u> as … (focus is on the self—reactive)
Perspective C: <u>Others</u>, the staff included, repeatedly perceive the <u>patient</u> as … (focus is on the other—active)
Perspective D: <u>Others</u>, the staff included, regularly experience <u>themselves</u> as … (focus is on the self—reactive)

This framework comprises the transference–countertransference configurations enacted between each patient and others, particularly the other patients and those members of staff most closely involved in their treatment within the clinical setting (Gordon, 1999; Gordon & Kirtchuk, 2008).

To summarise this key point: both participants in any interpersonal, self-other, interaction will have two basic types of experience. Each has an experience which consists of various perceptions of how the other is relating to the self: an active focus on the other's actions, behaviour, attitudes, and states of mind. In turn, as a response to these perceptions of the other, each person also has an experience of herself: a reactive focus on the self's actions, behaviour, attitudes, and states of mind. For example, to a perception of the other as critical and humiliating, the self may respond by feeling despair or, alternatively, by becoming offended or even running away. The whole forms a reliable and valid empirical structure to determine stable but dysfunctional patterns in relationships (Cierpka et al., 2007).

An in-depth exploration of these patterns helps to uncover the central, core interpersonal dynamics of the patient which are repeated time and again. Once the core dynamics are identified, it becomes possible to link past experiences in the patient's life with ways in which staff members may be unwittingly caught up in dramatic repetitions of those past patterns. From this material it is possible to hypothesise the significant internalised object relationships of the patient, the internal map of expected, desired, and feared relationships based on cumulative experience, and the manner in which these scenarios may influence external relationships on the ward. It is this largely unconscious pattern of relating, the transference–countertransference configuration, that is the focus of the ID four perspective consultation (as described by Stasch, Cierpka, Hillenbrand, & Schmal, 2002).

Identifying the negative to strengthen the positive

We have developed the ID protocol from the first version of the OPD Axis II (OPD Task Force, 2001) in order to specifically focus on the level of pathology and destructiveness of the group of patients with whom we work. In this sense, all of the cluster and item descriptions used in the ID consultation to elicit interpersonal patterns, including positive qualities such as "affirming" and "protecting", can be seen to have a latent, more negative dimension: for example, collusive, biased "affirming" and godfather-style "protecting". Our intention in interpreting the protocol in this way is not to apportion blame or ignore the real strengths of the patients and staff, but to use the consultation to identify what is maladaptive and problematic. This arises from our experience in a forensic setting where professionals are working on the edge of what is emotionally tolerable, where contact with catastrophic narratives is commonplace, and where "communication by impact" (Casement, 1985) is the rule. As mentioned above, in order to grasp the nature of clinical interactions in such an extreme setting and in work with such severely ill and dangerous patients, we have also used language from the Kleinian psychoanalytic perspective to modify some of the terms used in our versions of the cluster/item list and of the interpersonal circle (circumplex) (See Appendices One and Two). This language (for example, "destroying" instead of the more usual "hating", and "idealising" instead of "loving") fully encompasses an understanding of the challenges posed by the combination of psychosis, perversion, and psychopathic elements faced particularly but not exclusively by forensic mental health professionals. The aim of the consultation is always to elucidate the negative aspects of relating in order to strengthen the positive aspects.

The ID consultation: method

Administration

The interpersonal dynamics of any particular patient should be assessed at a multidisciplinary team meeting. Participants should include staff members who are personally involved with the patient, as well as a facilitator from outside the team who has expertise in formulating core relationship patterns. It is important that experiences are shared because, as we have outlined above, the patient may feel and behave differently towards various carers. The process is non-hierarchical as all perceptions and experiences are valid.

The consultation itself comprises four stages. The initial part is a presentation of background information, based on reports of the patient's past and current significant relationships, offending pathway and index offence (if relevant), before moving on to consider current relationship patterns with others and staff members. The reasons for the ID consultation are elicited at this stage in order to bring into focus the main problems inhibiting treatment and progress

(See Appendix I: the worksheet). Next, the interpersonal dynamics are determined using the four-perspective protocol. For each perspective the three or four most salient items are identified (See Appendix I: the cluster list). If there are two items identified in one cluster, it is best to choose the most accurate item. However if both items are equally present they should both be chosen, as this indicates the very strong relevance of the cluster. Regarding the first two perspectives (patient's perspective on others and on self), the clinical team must provide clear examples from statements the patient has made in the first person. Alternatively or additionally, a team member may conduct a consultation to the patient in order to obtain his views on the first two perspectives and offer an opportunity for the patient to contribute to her own recovery and overall treatment. All items that are selected on the protocol must have clear evidence, based on statements and examples. A basic formulation is then produced which attempts to construct a working hypothesis linking the four perspectives in the form of a maladaptive vicious cycle. Such a cycle describes a joint narrative of how patient and staff construct and experience their core relationships in the here-and-now. Next an expanded formulation is developed which links the emerging current interpersonal dynamics with past relationship patterns, including the index offence. Finally the treatment strategy is reviewed in the light of the ID formulations.

Time

We currently undertake this process in two meetings of up to one hour each. In the first meeting the first three stages—history, cluster/item selection, and basic formulation—take place; between the meetings the formulation is elaborated, usually by the facilitator of the ID consultation; and the second meeting is for the review of clinical care, risk assessment, and management based on a discussion of the expanded formulation. However, more complex cases may need additional meetings to understand and work through the implications of the formulations. The ID consultation process may be repeated every six months, preferably before the patient's care planning meeting.

Setting

It is strongly recommended that the ID consultation be used in a group setting involving various members of the MDT. In our experience the presence of professionals from three or more disciplines within an MDT such as doctors, nurses, art therapists, occupational therapist, psychologist, or social worker is most useful in collecting a sufficient amount of clinical information related to staff-patient interactions, some of which might otherwise be ignored or considered trivial (for example, a casual conversation with a health care assistant during escorted leave), in order to identify the most significant patterns of dysfunctional interpersonal relationships.

However, we have increasingly found that a brief form of the ID consultation (perspectives A and B) can also be used by individual practitioners to improve the overall assessment of patients in routine clinical work, although obviously the views of other team members will not be included in this application. Nevertheless, working individually with a patient to elicit his views on how others are perceived and how the patient responds offers patients an opportunity to assume a more active role in contributing to his treatment, in enhancing staff awareness as well as in learning about himself. It also demonstrates authentic staff interest and concern regarding how patients experience their interpersonal world. Some patients might be able to go even further and begin to develop an empathic understanding of staff by completing perspectives C and D. In effect, this individual mode of the ID consultation serves both as a focal point of the therapeutic alliance and as a springboard for a mentalization-based treatment approach which enhances patients' capacity to be curious about the existence and functioning of their own and others' minds. A format for this individualised approach may be found in Appendix III.

User qualifications

The ID consultation is designed to help all mental health professionals working within multidisciplinary teams. It is especially important for those who have continuing contact with patients and who make routine mental state assessments within a clinical setting, as well as trainees who are specialising in a relevant field. It is vital that senior clinicians take a lead in organising ID meetings and arranging for background information on the referred patient to be available.

We also advise that MDT members regularly utilise the protocol within their setting in order to obtain a high degree of proficiency in arriving at a formulation which can contribute to care plans and risk assessment.

Formulations: basic and expanded

The formulation should consist of two separate yet linked narrative strands. A basic formulation uses information on the four perspectives derived from the highlighted clusters and items on the protocol which have emerged in the consultation. Therefore, the formulation begins with (A) the patient repeatedly perceives others as … (B) and in response, the patient experiences himself as … continuing on to (C) others repeatedly perceive the patient as … (D) and in response experience themselves as … So for example, the patient repeatedly perceives others as domineering, imposing, and abandoning, and in response the patient experiences himself as behaving as if he knows best and cutting off contact. Consequently, others (the staff) repeatedly perceive the patient as insisting on his position and keeping up a barrier, which leads them to experience themselves as either domineering and imposing or giving up in despair. In effect this simply reinforces the patient's original perception that others are controlling and abandoning.

In collecting evidence for each perspective, it is important to identify features in both the here and now relationships within the clinical setting as well as in past experiences of the patient. The four perspectives often describe a dysfunctional cycle that repeats relationship patterns from past to present (see Figure 1 below). It is important to re-emphasise that the consultation is concerned with these dysfunctional aspects of relating because, although they are precisely the ones which are most difficult to bear, to attend to and to think about, they also contain very

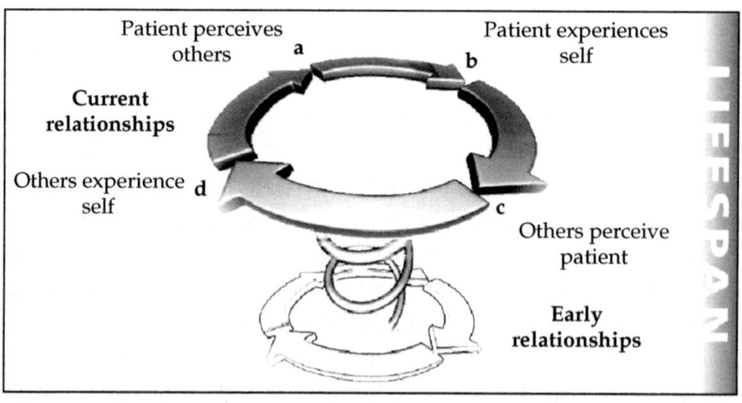

Figure 1. Transference–countertransference.

significant information about the characteristic functioning of the patient's mind as expressed in his social relationships.

A further, expanded formulation includes a more detailed emotional narrative of the patient's core repertoire of relationship patterns as they have developed in the course of the patient's life, especially with significant early caretakers as illustrated in the diagram above. The presence of an appropriately trained practitioner will significantly facilitate the construction of this more comprehensive formulation. The key task is to show how the patient's perceptions of others may involve misattributions of characteristics belonging either to the patient or to important figures in the patient's past, who in turn respond automatically to the impact of these attributions. For example a patient who cannot tolerate feelings of intense guilt may behave in such a way so as to aggravate and so draw criticisms from staff, who accordingly take on the role perhaps of a highly critical parent. Subsequently, the patient will naturally feel guilty for upsetting staff or rebel against unjustifiable criticism which might make staff even more authoritarian. In this manner the patient's own guilt seems to be dramatised in the form of rebukes, now emanating from a person in the external world. Conversely, staff may also contribute to the dysfunctional relationship as a result of their own make up or other unresolved conflicts , for example, conflict within the staff team. An important aim of the expanded formulation is to illuminate the presenting interpersonal problems which initiated the consultation and those which might increase risk, including the interpersonal dynamics represented by the index offence. The formulation is accessible to all professionals and provides a framework within which each professional can act in accordance with her own way of working. However, the process of discussion itself is as important as the formulation.

Implications for care plans and risk assessment

An important aim of the consultation should be to allow the formulation to inform future care plans, risk assessment, and the overall treatment and management of the patient. The implications of the core interpersonal dynamics may cast light on how best to manage the patient's care. For example, one may consider whether, due to a tendency to perceive the patient as "special", one is caught up in making allowances that further the patient's grandiosity or feelings of entitlement. A practical consideration would be to review any special arrangements in place for that patient. Another example may be where a patient is allowed too much independence because of a difficulty in managing the level of despair and hopelessness the patient engenders in staff. In this sense the staff may be enacting an earlier relationship where caregivers effectively abandoned the patient and left him to fend for himself. All of these situations may have an impact on risk of further offending, or recreate scenarios that are similar to the index offence and so need careful consideration and management.

The interpersonal circle (circumplex)

The interpersonal circumplex (Appendix II) is a two dimensional visual representation, a circle drawn around horizontal and vertical axes, which allows one to plot the core relationship interactions between a subject and the significant others in her life. The cluster/item list is based on this map of characteristics which can describe interpersonal relationships. As mentioned above in the theoretical and empirical review, the horizontal axis traditionally denotes a range from extremely negative to extremely positive positions in regard to proximity/affiliation ("destroying"/"idealising"); and the vertical axis similarly charts a spectrum of positions in regard to control ("allowing (total) independence"/"(totally) controlling"). The circle can also be viewed as composed of four quadrants, marked by the relationship characteristics (clusters) indicated at right angles. At the mid-point of each quadrant, along the perimeter of the circle, further descriptions of interpersonal interactions may be placed which are blends of the two clusters located at the quadrant's boundaries. For example, in the lower left quadrant of the active circle, bounded by "controlling" and "destroying", "blaming" is located at the intermediate point on the basis that "blaming" contains modified aspects of both "controlling" and "destroying" clusters. The quadrant structure will be described in more detail below.

Although two circles are illustrated, they should be understood as showing two layers of the circumplex map, active and reactive (Benjamin 1996), which together portray different aspects of the interpersonal relationship. As mentioned, the active layer always refers to how the subject, whether patient or staff member, actively perceives and interprets the actions, behaviours, attitudes, and states of mind of the other. The reactive layer refers to how the subject accordingly responds to these perceptions.

The active circle: items 1–16

The vertical axis of the active circle is "allowing independence" versus "controlling", and the horizontal axis is "destroying" versus "idealising". Starting from the top of the circle, these four points mark key stages in a journey through the clusters divided into four quadrants. The first quadrant ranges from "allowing independence" to "idealising" with "affirming" at the midpoint. The offer of freedom perceived in the "allowing independence" cluster may amount to a neglectful ignoring ("treating as self-sufficiently independent") which echoes the "destroying"—"abandoning" clusters in quadrant 4 to its left; or, moving clockwise, it may become a collusive indulgence expressing an extremely accepting and positive view. This becomes "idealising" when the other is viewed as treating the subject as special and exceptional, leading to an over-estimation and inability to see any negative aspects. The second quadrant moves from "idealising" to "controlling" by way of "protecting", The milder form of "protecting", closer to "idealising", is expressed as "attending to and caring for in every way"; whereas the form influenced more by the "controlling" cluster at the bottom of the quadrant is described as a mafia "godfather"-like "instructing and patronising". The second quadrant ends with "controlling" which reflects varied facets of ruthless domination. The third quadrant moves from "controlling" to "destroying" with "blaming" at the mid-point, the latter expressed first as accusations in a more "controlling" mode and then in behaviour which becomes more destructively "putting down and humiliating". At its extreme the third quadrant becomes the "intimidating" and "attacking" behaviour of the "destroying" cluster. The fourth quadrant moves from "destroying" to "allowing independence" with "abandoning" situated at mid-point. The second item in the "destroying" cluster is "rejecting and excluding", a more subtle form of "destroying" contact which shares aspects of the adjacent "abandoning" cluster . "Abandoning" then leads us back to the top of the circle, returning to the neglectful freedom of "allowing independence" with which we began.

There are eight clusters each of which includes two descriptive items. It may seem that there is little differentiation between the two items, but as just indicated by the examples characterising our journey around the perimeter of the active circumplex, they are designed to denote subtle differences influenced by their positions in relation to the four key points on the axes, as well as to neighbouring clusters at the midpoints. Once again focusing on the first cluster, the perception of "allowing independence" might be closer to "abandoning" (and the "destroying" cluster of quadrant 4) or, alternatively, to "affirming" (and the "idealising" cluster of quadrant 1).

The reactive circle: items 17–32

The vertical axis of the reactive circle is "asserting" versus "submitting", and the horizontal axis is "recoiling" versus "reactive idealising". The first quadrant moves from "asserting" to "reactive idealising" with "disclosing" at midpoint. "Asserting" might be expressed through "defying and opposing" behaviour which, by keeping the responding self distant from others, is coloured by the "isolating"/"recoiling" clusters characterising quadrant 4 on its left; or, moving clockwise towards the "disclosing" and "reactive idealising" clusters of quadrant 1, self responds by "insisting on his position", imbued with "over revealing and intrusive" behaviour and increasing over involvement and merging with the idealised other. The second quadrant covers "reactive idealising" to "submitting" with "depending" at the midpoint. "Depending" is expressed by "over relying on" as it approaches "reactive idealising" of the other and, changing its tone, becomes increasingly parasitical and passive as it nears the "submitting" cluster at the bottom of quadrant 2. The third quadrant, moving from "submitting" to "recoiling", represents how "the worm turns". From abject submission the self begins to develop a "hurt and touchy", increasingly "indignant and self-justifying" stance, which ultimately leads to "recoiling" from the other. "Recoiling" condenses alternating fight/flight responses: like a recoiling rifle, movement can be aggressively toward ("showing disgust") or away from ("running away") the other. Finally, the fourth quadrant begins with the "recoiling" cluster, continues to "isolating" at midpoint and completes the circle with "asserting". Bordering the flight aspect of the "recoiling" cluster, "isolating" is expressed by "running away". As it approaches the top of quadrant 4, "isolating" begins to reflect aspects of "cutting off contact", the "defying and opposing" of the "asserting" cluster with which our journey started.

As in the active circle, each of the eight reactive clusters comprise two items which denote subtle differences influenced by their positions in relation to the four key clusters on the axes and to adjacent midpoint clusters. Therefore, the "asserting" response at the top of the circumplex may be closer to "keeping up a barrier" as expressed by the "isolating" "recoiling" clusters of the preceding fourth quadrant; or, alternatively, "asserting" becomes more insistent and absorbing as it approaches the "disclosing"—"reactive idealising" clusters of the first quadrant.

Consulting to chaos

The next two chapters provide respectively a practical and a theoretical context for understanding the vital role that regular use of ID consultations can play in mental health settings. Maja Turcan (Chapter One) describes a qualitative research project which sought to explore clinicians' experiences of their work in a forensic service and shows how the ID consultation can offer significant help to professionals in managing both their clinical and organisational dilemmas. Gill McGauley (Chapter Two) reviews the literature on attachment theory and mentalization and discovers some cogent links between these substantial, evidence-based therapeutic orientations and the ID consultation. We then give a number of examples of the ID consultation in action. Maggie McAlister (Chapter Three) shows how subtle, perverse enactments—and their effects on the functioning of the multidisciplinary team—can be elicited and contained by the ID consultation process. Ronald Doctor (Chapter Four) adapts the method to reflect on a case of homicide and emphasises how surprisingly easy it is for professionals to downplay serious violence. Amber Fossey, Gabriel Kirtchuk, and David Reiss (Chapter Five) consider the importance of the ID consultation in effective risk assessment and management. Richard Church, Gabriel Kirtchuk, and David Reiss (Chapter Six) demonstrate the relevance of the ID consultation for staff working in the fraught, multi-agency community setting of child protection, clearly indicating that the ID approach has a contribution to make well beyond the in-patient forensic psychiatric hospital where it was developed. Aikaterini Papaspirou and Jose Maret (Chapter Seven) conclude the case studies with the psychoanalytic and quintessentially forensic classic: an ID consultation to Oedipus. The last two chapters of the book again widen the focus. John Gordon, Richard Ingram, and Gabriel Kirtchuk (Chapter Eight) trace the development of an MSc level course in psychodynamic approaches to individual, group, and organisational dynamics which we would consider a requisite training for prospective interpersonal dynamics consultants. Then John Gordon and Gabriel Kirtchuk (Conclusion) elaborate a key point from the Introduction and emphasise the function of the ID consultation as a crucial form of patient-centred reflective practice which should be an indispensable priority in the minds of senior managers in all mental health, prison/probation, and community social services. For without it patients, staff, and organisations inevitably go adrift and sometimes crash. At the end of the volume in Appendix III, Beate Schumacher offers an adapted ID consultation for use with individuals rather than teams.

We would like to acknowledge the contributions of Maggie McAlister and David Reiss to some of the material used in this chapter regarding the history and administration of the ID consultation, earlier versions of which appeared in Gordon and Kirtchuk (2008), Reiss and Kirtchuk (2009), and Kirtchuk, Gordon, McAlister, and Reiss (2013).

References

Allport, G. W. (1937). *Personality: A Psychological Interpretation*. New York: Henry Holt.

American Psychiatric Association. (2013). *Diagnostic and Statistical Manual of Mental Disorders (5th Edition)*. Washington: APA Press.

Armstrong, D., & Rustin, M. (2014) *Social Defences Against Anxiety: Explorations in a Paradigm*. London: Karnac.

Bateman, A. W. & Fonagy, P. (2004). *Psychotherapy for Borderline Personality Disorder: Mentalization-Based Treatment*. Oxford: Oxford University Press.

Beckett, S. (1956). *Malone Dies*. In: *Three Novels: Molloy, Malone Dies, The Unnamable*. New York, NY: The Grove Press.

Benjamin, L. S. (1996). *Interpersonal Diagnosis and Treatment of Personality Disorders*. New York, NY: Guilford Press.

Bion, W. R. (1959). Attacks on linking. *International Journal of Psychoanalysis, 40*: 308–315. Also in: *Second Thoughts: Selected Papers on Psychoanalysis*. London: Maresfield Reprints, 1967/1984.

Bion, W. R. (1961). *Experiences in Groups*. London: Tavistock.

Bion, W. R. (1962/1984). *Learning From Experience*. London: Maresfield Library.

Bion, W. R. (1970/1984). *Attention and Interpretation*. London: Maresfield Library.

Bion, W. R. (1979). Making the best of a bad job. In: *Clinical Seminars and Four Papers* (pp. 247–257). Abingdon: Fleetwood Press.

Birtchnell, J. (1993). *How Humans Relate: A New Interpersonal Theory*. Westport, CT: Praeger.

Blackburn, R. (1998). Criminality and the interpersonal circle in forensic psychiatric patients. *Criminal Justice and Behaviour, 25*: 155–176.

Bowlby, J. (1969). *Attachment and Loss, Volume I. Attachment*. London: The Hogarth Press and The Institute of Psychoanalysis.

Bowlby, J. (1973). *Attachment and Loss, Volume II. Separation: Anxiety and Anger*. London: The Hogarth Press and The Institute of Psychoanalysis.

Campling, P., Davies, S., & Farquharson, G. (Eds.). (2004). *From Toxic Institutions to Therapeutic Environments: Residential Settings in Mental Health Services*. London: Gaskell.

Casement, P. (1985). *On Learning from the Patient*. London: Brunner-Routledge.

Cierpka, M., Grande, T., Rudolf, G., von der Tann, M., Stasch, M. & OPD Task Force. (2007). The operationalized psychodynamic diagnostics system: Clinical relevance, reliability and validity. *Psychopathology, 40*: 209–220.

Dahlbender, R. W., Rudolf, G., & OPD Task Force. (2006). Psychic structure and mental functioning: Current research on the reliable measurement and clinical validity of operationalised psychodynamic diagnostics (OPD) system. In: PDM Task Force (Ed.), *Psychodynamic Diagnostic Manual* (pp. 615–662). Silver Spring: Alliance of Psychoanalytic Organizations.

Freud, S. (1933). Why War? In: *The Standard Edition of the Complete Psychological Works of Sigmund Freud. Volume XXII* (pp. 195–216). London: The Hogarth Press and The Institute of Psychoanalysis.

Gordon, J. (1994). Bion's post-*Experiences in Groups* thinking on groups: A clinical example of -K. In: V. L. Schermer & M. Pines (Eds.), *Ring of Fire: Primitive Affects and Object Relations in Group Psychotherapy* (pp. 107–127). London: Routledge.

Gordon, J. (1999). Paula Heimann's question and group analysis. *Psychoanalytic Psychotherapy, 13*: 107–116.

Gordon, J. (2004). Review of *Dangerous Patients: A Psychodynamic Approach to Risk Assessment and Management. Psychoanalytic Psychotherapy, 18*: 347–351.

Gordon, J. (2011). Some neglected clinical material from Bion's *Experiences in Groups*. In: C. Mawson (Ed.), *Bion Today* (pp. 330–346). The New Library of Psychoanalysis. London: Routledge.

Gordon, J., & Kirtchuk, G. (Eds.). (2008). *Psychic Assaults and Frightened Clinicians: Countertransference in Forensic Settings*. London: Karnac.

Gordon, J., Harding, S., Miller, C., and Xenitides, K. (2005). X-treme group analysis: On the countertransference edge in inpatient work with forensic patients. *Group Analysis, 38*: 409–426. Also in: J. Gordon, & G. Kirtchuk, (Eds.). (2008). *Psychic Assaults and Frightened Clinicians: Countertransference in Forensic Settings* (pp. 41–61). London: Karnac.

Gosling, R. (1968). What is transference? In: J. Sutherland (Ed.), *The Psychoanalytic Approach* (pp. 1–10). London: Bailliere, Tindal, and Cassell.

Greenburg, J. R., & Mitchell, S. A. (1983). *Object Relations in Psychoanalytic Theory*. Cambridge, Mass: Harvard University Press.

Gross, S., Stasch, M., Schmal, H., Hillenbrand, E., & Cierpka, M. (2007). Changes in mental representations of relational behaviour in depressive patients. *Psychotherapy Research, 17*: 522–534.

Guttman, L. C. (1996). Order analysis of correlation matrices. In: R. B. Cattle (Ed.), *Handbook of Multivariate Experimental Psychology* (pp. 439–458). Chicago, IL: Rand McNall.

Hinshelwood, R. D. (1994). Attacks on the reflective space: Containing primitive emotional states. In: V. L. Schermer & M. Pines (Eds.), *Ring of Fire: Primitive Affects and Object Relations in Group Psychotherapy* (pp. 86–106). London: Routledge.

Hinshelwood, R. D. (1999). The difficult patient: the role of "scientific psychiatry" in understanding patients with chronic schizophrenia or personality disorder. *British Journal of Psychiatry, 174*: 187–190.

Hinshelwood, R. D. (2004). *Suffering Insanity: Psychoanalytic Essays on Psychosis*. London: Brunner-Routledge.

Hinshelwood, R. D., & Skogstad, W. (Eds.). (2000). *Observing Organisations: anxiety, Defence and Culture in Health Care*. London: Taylor & Francis.

Hinshelwood, R. D., & Skogstad, W. (2002). Irradiated by distress: Observing psychic pain in health-care organisations. *Psychoanalytic Psychotherapy, 16*: 110–124.

Hirschhorn, L. (1995). *The Workplace Within: Psychodynamics of Organisational Life*. Cambridge, Mass: MIT Press.

Hoffman, I., & Gill, M. M. (1988). A scheme for coding the patient's experience of the relationship with the therapist (PERT): Some applications, extensions and comparisons. In: H. Dahl, H. Kachele, & H. Thoma (Eds.), *Psychoanalytic Process Research Strategies* (pp. 67–98). Berlin: Springer.

Horowitz, M. (1991). *Personal Schemas and Maladaptive Interpersonal Behavior*. Chicago, Il: University of Chicago Press.

Hughes, T. (1969). *Seneca's Oedipus*. London: Faber & Faber.

Jaques, E. (1955). Social systems as a defence against persecutory and depressive anxiety: In: M. Klein, P. Heimann, & R. Money-Kyrle (Eds.), *New Directions in Psycho-Analysis* (pp. 478–498). London: Tavistock.

Joseph, B. (1989). *Psychic Equilibrium and Psychic Change: Selected Papers of Betty Joseph*. E. B. Spillius & M. Feldman (Eds.). The New Library of Psychoanalysis. London: Routledge.

Kirtchuk, G., Gordon, J., McAlister, M., & Reiss, D. (2013). *Interpersonal Dynamics Consultation: A Manual for Clinicians*. London: www.lulu.com Press.

Klein, M. (1946). Notes on some schizoid mechanisms. *International Journal of Psychoanalysis, 27*: 99–110. Also in: *Writings 1: Love, Guilt and Reparation* (pp. 370–419). London: Hogarth Press, 1975.

Klein, M. (1955). On identification. In: M. Klein, P. Heimann & R. Money-Kyrle (Eds.), *New Directions in Psycho-Analysis* (pp. 309–345). London: Tavistock.

Leary, T. (1957). *Interpersonal Diagnosis of Personality: A Functional Theory and Methodology for Personality Evaluation*. New York, NY: Ronald Press.

Luborsky, L., & Crits-Christoph, P. (1990). *Understanding Transference*. New York, NY: Basic.

Meltzer, D. (1992). *The Claustrum: An Investigation of Claustrophobic Phenomena*. London: The Clunie Press.

Menzies Lyth, I. (1960). A case study in the functioning of social systems as a defence against anxiety. *Human Relations, 13*: 95–121. Reprinted in: *Containing Anxiety in Institutions: Selected Essays, Volume 1* (pp. 26–44). London: Free Association Books, 1988.

Money-Kyrle, R. (1956). Normal countertransference and some of its deviations. *International Journal of Psychoanalysis, 37*: 360–366.

Murray, H. A. (1938). *Explorations in Personality*. Oxford: Oxford University Press.

Ogden, T. H. (1982). *Projective Identification and Psychoanalytic Technique*. New York, NY: Jason Aronson.

OPD Task Force. (2001). *Operationalized Psychodynamic Diagnostics: Foundations and Manual*. Gottingen: Hogrefe and Huber.

OPD Task Force. (2008). *Operationalized Psychodynamic Diagnostics 2: Manual of Diagnosis and Treatment Planning*. Cambridge, Mass: Hogrefe and Huber.

Pick, I. B. (1985). Working through in the countertransference. *International Journal of Psychoanalysis, 66*: 157–166.

Platonov, A. (1999/2001). *Happy Moscow*. London: The Harvill Press.

Racker, H. (1968). *Transference and Countertransference*. London: Maresfield Reprints.

Reiss, D., & Kirtchuk, G. (2009). Interpersonal dynamics and multidisciplinary teamwork. *Advances in Psychiatric Treatment, 15*: 462–469.

Rosenfeld, H. (1987). *Impasse and Interpretation*. London: Tavistock/Routledge.

Schaefer, E. S. (1965). Configuration analysis of children's reports of parent behavior. *Journal of Consulting Psychology, 29*: 552–557.

Schore, A. (2002). Effects of a secure attachment relationship on right brain development, affect regulation and infant mental health. *Infant Mental Health Journal, 22*: 7–66.

Segal, H. (1986). *The Work of Hanna Segal: A Kleinian Approach to Clinical Practice*. London: Free Association Books.

Sodre, I. (2015). *Imaginary Existences: A Psychoanalytic Exploration of Phantasy, Fiction, Dreams and Daydreams*. The New Library of Psychoanalysis. London: Routledge.

Spillius, E. B. (Ed.). (1988a). *Melanie Klein Today, 1: Mainly Theory*. The New Library of Psychoanalysis. London: Routledge.

Spillius, E. B. (Ed.). (1988b). *Melanie Klein Today, 2: Mainly Practice*. The New Library of Psychoanalysis. London: Routledge.

Spillius, E. B., & O'Shaughnessy, E. (Ed.). (2011). *Projective Identification: The Fate of a Concept*. The New Library of Psychoanalysis. London: Routledge.

Stasch, M. (2004). Interpersonal tuning in inpatient psychotherapy: A clinical approach based on the operationalised psychodynamic diagnostics (OPD). 34th annual meeting of the Society for Psychotherapy Research, Weimar.

Stasch, M., Cierpka, M., Hillenbrand, E., & Schmal, H. (2002). Assessing reenactment in inpatient psychodynamic therapy. *Psychotherapy Research, 12*: 355–368.

Steiner, J. (1993). *Psychic Retreats*. London: Routledge.

Strupp, H., & Binder, J. (1984). *Psychotherapy in a New Key: A Guide to Time-Limited Dynamic Psychotherapy*. New York, NY: Basic.

Sullivan, H. S. (1953). *The Interpersonal Theory of Psychiatry*. New York, NY: Norton.

Treasaden, I. (2003). Assessment of violence in medium-secure units. In: R. Doctor (Ed.), *Dangerous Patients: A Psychodynamic Approach to Risk Assessment and Management. Psychoanalytic Psychotherapy* (pp. 21–31). London: Karnac.

Weiss, J., & Sampson, H. (1986). *The Psychoanalytic Process: Theory, Clinical Observation and Empirical Research*. New York, NY: Guilford Press.

World Health Organization. (1994). *International Classification of Diseases 10*. www.who.int/whosis/icd10/ last accessed 1 March 2016.

CHAPTER ONE

Researching chaos and generating meanings: a qualitative study

Maja Turcan

> Qualitative methods are particularly useful to illuminate how individuals perceive social systems and how those social systems function in a natural context. It might be argued that this is particularly important in the multidisciplinary setting and way of working. (Wix, Riordan, & Humphreys, 2005, p. 207)

The book from which this quotation was taken does not have any chapter about, or using, qualitative methodology. It is an edited book called *Multidisciplinary Working in Forensic Mental Health Care*. There are in fact few studies using qualitative methodology in forensic mental health. There may be many reasons for the paucity of qualitative methodological approaches in studying the experience of working in multidisciplinary teams in forensic settings. For example quantitative research is more familiar, may be easier to undertake and may be preferred by researchers, and some consider qualitative research to be less scientific and more difficult to replicate. However, it is an approach that provides the opportunity to explore in depth the experiences of a group of individuals in a particular context, especially the meanings individuals attribute to their subjective perceptions of their experiences, which in turn can lead to unexpected findings worthy of further research and development. There are a number of qualitative research methodologies. This study used Interpretative Phenomenological Analysis (IPA) to analyse the data that was collected using semi-structured interviews.

The aim of the study described in this chapter was to explore how participants as members of a multidisciplinary team make sense of working in a forensic setting with mentally disordered offenders. By taking account of the specific context in which events occur, it set out to explore the perspectives of the participants as clinicians; how they organise their thinking and communication about their work, training, and patients; and to what extent the clinical management and the organisational structures foster communication and support.

Methodology

Design

A small group qualitative study was conducted using a semi-structured interview format and IPA methodology for data analysis developed by Smith (1995) and Smith, Flowers, and Larkin (2009) and used and described by others (Reid, Flowers, & Larkin, 2005; Shaw, 2001).

Sample

The sample comprised seven participants. Smith (2004) suggested that if a detailed case-by-case analysis is being carried out, then a small sample of about five to ten participants is appropriate. IPA is specifically conducive to examining a small sample in detail; it was particularly suitable for this study that used purposive sampling, which means deliberately choosing a relatively homogeneous group of participants for whom the research question was meaningful.

Participants

The research participants in this study were senior clinical members of staff who, in addition to their core training and responsibilities, have undertaken training in the use of the Operationalised Psychodynamic Diagnostics (OPD) that offers a framework that seeks to generate a shared formulation, understanding, and communication within the team of the psychological processes underlying patients' interpersonal difficulties. This group of professionals were involved in regular clinical meetings/seminars using the Interpersonal Dynamics (ID) consultation, based on Axis II of the OPD, to formulate patients' interpersonal interactions.

All the participants had thereby been systematically exposed to another framework of conceptual thinking in addition to their core training. This allowed the participants to make a choice, when discussing their thoughts and views about patients, between the frameworks of their core professions, the framework offered by OPD/ID, and any combination of the two.

Description of participants

Participant one (Ms A) is a female nurse in her thirties with seven years post qualifying experience, and was finishing a Masters degree in organisational consultancy (psychoanalytic approaches). Ms A had extensive experience of face-to-face forensic nursing in acute, high secure and medium secure psychiatric settings. She also had some four years experience of supervising ward based nurses.

Participant two (Ms B) is a female drama therapist in her late thirties with ten years post qualifying experience. Ms B had completed a psychoanalytic training in the previous year but worked in the forensic unit as drama therapist. More recently she had started to supervise drama therapists as well as professionals from other core disciplines.

Participant three (Dr C) is a male consultant psychiatrist and psychoanalyst, sixty years old, with many years of previous experience as a psychiatrist and about twelve years of working in a forensic unit as a psychoanalyst. Most of his work consisted of supervising and teaching members of Multidisciplinary Teams (MDT), leading reflective practice for staff and some direct patient contact. The direct patient contact consisted of assessments for treatment and for the purpose of contributing to teams' deliberations and formulation when they felt stuck.

Participant four (Ms D) is a female art therapist with at least twelve years experience of working in various forensic settings. She is in her early forties. Most of Ms D's experience was that of direct patient clinical work, and she had extensive experience for the previous eight years of supervising staff within her own profession as well as nursing staff. She was the head of her department. Ms D was, at the time of the study, undergoing psychoanalytic training.

Participant five (Dr E) is a male specialist registrar in forensic psychiatry. He is in his mid thirties. Dr E trained abroad and worked there as a psychiatrist for five years. He has worked as a forensic psychiatrist in England. He has daily direct contact with patients.

Participant six (Dr F) is a male consultant psychologist and group analyst. He is in his early sixties. Dr F had worked in a forensic setting for the previous ten years. Most of his work consisted of staff teaching, supervision, and reflective practice. He also undertook some direct patient clinical work.

Participant seven (Dr G) is a male consultant forensic psychiatrist with eight years experience as a consultant. He is in his early forties. Dr G was involved in postgraduate psychiatric training and research in addition to his clinical work.

Setting

The research was carried out in an inpatient NHS medium secure unit. In this service all patients are on compulsory treatment orders with an average length of stay of about three years with a range of a few months to eighteen years. Most patients are in the service because of serious interpersonal violence, including homicide. The most common diagnoses in the adult services are psychotic illnesses such as schizophrenia and its variants, affective disorders and personality disorders. Sometimes these diagnoses may exist in combination and may be complicated further with substance misuse and borderline learning disability. Many of the patients have also come from adverse circumstances that may include significant trauma or abuse.

Most patients are well known to their team as a result of their long inpatient stay. The nursing staff, understandably, are expected to have the most intimate knowledge of the patients as they spend the most time with them.

The clinical structure of the service comprises a consultant forensic psychiatrist led multidisciplinary team, consisting of junior medical staff, psychologist, occupational therapist, art therapist, and nurses. There are also teachers, physical instructors, and dieticians available to the team. The organisational clinical structures consist of regular weekly multidisciplinary clinical team meetings known as Ward Rounds, where the MDT meets to discuss the individual member's involvement with patients and their thoughts about them, and where the future care plan decisions about the patient are made. The patient is invited to attend the ward round. There is a six-monthly Care Plan Approach (CPA) meeting where long term plans are discussed with patients and their therapists and carers. Most MDTs have regular, usually weekly, "reflective practice" and some form of supervision. Reflective practice consists of a protected time and setting that staff may access in a group format, facilitated by an experienced psychoanalytic psychotherapist, to discuss patients, concerns, and feelings engendered by the work. The sessions are not structured, and staff are at liberty to raise whatever topics they choose.

Materials

Semi-structured interview schedule

The semi-structured interview consisted of four broad questions, focusing on three main areas: experience of working in a forensic setting, the participants' experience of being a member of the MDT and of its functioning, and preparation for the job. The topics to be explored were the result of literature review and reflection on clinical and supervision experience of the author. The questions guided the interview but were sufficiently flexible to allow the participants to raise questions and to answer the questions in the way that they felt was relevant (Smith, 1995). The interviews were conducted with relatively few prompts from the interviewer in order to encourage and to elicit the participants' own experience.

The questions were as follows:

A: **What is it like to work with forensic patients?**
This section focused on the participant's experience of working with forensic patients in the forensic setting. Prompts:
1. What led you to work in a forensic setting?
2. Was it a choice or circumstances?
3. What were/are your expectations?

(e.g., Aiyegbusi & Tuck, 2008; Happel, Pinikahana, & Martin, 2003).

B: **What is it like to work with forensic patients as a member of an MDT**
This section focused on the participant's experience of working as a member of the MDT. Prompts:
1. How do you understand your role as a member of a MDT?

2. How does it contribute to your work with forensic patients, being a member of a MDT?
3. What does it mean in this setting working as a member of a MDT?
4. Do you feel that you are a member of a MDT?

(e.g., Liberman, Hilty, Drake, & Tsang, 2001).

C: **In what way do the core trainings and experiences prepare the members of the MDT for work in a forensic setting?**

This section focused on the participant's training and experiences, how they felt they applied them in their daily work and how they prepared them for what they actually do. Prompts:

1. What skills from your training would you draw on trying to understand or manage patients' behaviour?
2. Are there any specific tools or interactions that you find particularly useful?
3. In what way has your own core training prepared you to understand and manage the patients' behaviour in a forensic setting?

(e.g., Mason & Carton, 2002).

D: **What are the existing structures that are available to the MDT to do the job of understanding and managing patients' behaviour?**

This section focused on the participants' experience of the existing organisational and clinical structures that offer "thinking" spaces for understanding patients' behaviours and conflicts and the impact these structures would have on the experience of managing patients. Prompts:

1. Where do the members of the MDT meet to discuss patients' difficulties and the impact they have on behaviour?
2. Do those meetings do the job of [facilitating] understanding of patients' interpersonal difficulties?
3. How do members of MDT communicate in these meetings?

(e.g., Humphreys, 2005).

The semi-structured interview schedule was constructed to open the interview with a broad open question as an introduction. The questions that followed had to be presented in such an order that was logical and facilitated the participants' accounts. The order of the questions and the prompts were discussed with colleagues.

In the interviews prompts were used infrequently as the areas explored were considered relevant to the participants, and they needed little prompting to talk either about their own experiences or about the issues raised by the four main questions. Thus, most of the same issues were covered from participants' individual viewpoints.

Interpretative Phenomenological Analysis (IPA)

An in-depth analysis of subjective experiences of individuals was carried out.

Using the IPA the participants are trying to make sense of their world while the researcher is trying to make sense of the participants' world. This is made complicated by the researcher's own conceptions which are inevitable and necessary for the process of interpretation. There is thus a two stage interpretative process going on. The meanings that the process is seeking are in both the social and the personal world of the participant. IPA assumes connection between the way people talk and think and their emotional world. Consequently, interpretation implies that the researcher interprets the participant's inner world, mental and emotional state, from what they say and how they say it.

The use of language in interpreting is seen as important as it is assumed to contribute to the communication of what the participant is thinking. The link between the form and the content of the language is assumed to be present and is thus a part of the analysis. The linguistic element is seen as contributory but not as central as it is, for example, in discourse analysis (e.g., Willig, 2008).

The phenomenon under investigation here was the range of participants' subjective experiences within the setting in which they occur. The setting was a forensic psychiatric service. According to Giorgi and Giorgi:

> to study a particular phenomenon, a situation is sought in which individuals have first-hand experiences that they can describe as they actually took place in their life. The aim is to capture as closely as possible the way in which the phenomenon is experienced within the context in which the experience takes place. (Giorgi & Giorgi, 2008, p. 28)

IPA is phenomenological and its "main currency" (Smith & Osborn, 2008, p. 53) is the individual's experience and the meaning it holds for that individual. IPA is an inductive approach; the research process is dynamic involving the researcher and it accepts that the researcher is unlikely to approach the task from a wholly atheoretical stance and he or she is likely to bring prior knowledge and assumptions to the perception of the subject matter. This is considered legitimate provided it is fully acknowledged. IPA is specifically a psychological research method conducive to examining a small sample in detail, exploring how participants respond and what sense they make of a particular experience. IPA research explores the reflection that the participants engage in about an experience or about a part of their life.

Larkin and colleagues describe IPA as "accessible, flexible and applicable" (Larkin, Watts, & Clifton, 2006, p. 103) but they warn that flexibility does not stand for lack of rigour. The study followed the flexible, but rigorously reported, procedure proposed by Smith, Jarman, and Osborn (1999) and Smith, Flowers, & Larkin (2009).

Procedure for data collection

The study was presented by the author in the clinical OPD/ID seminar. Members were informed that those who were interested to participate in the study would be approached individually by the author with more information about the research and what exactly would be required of them. Given that the recruiting for the project was done in the seminar, and that the potential group from which the participants could be drawn was relatively small, only a partial confidentiality could be guaranteed. The participants may have inferred who else would be likely to participate in the research project. The participants were aware of this.

Any research exploring clinical practice may give rise to concerns that the participant staff's practice is under scrutiny. It was made clear to all the participating staff that their responses would be confidential and that no individual responses would be disclosed to anyone.

The researcher was asking her colleagues to discuss matters that could be difficult. Reflecting on the experience of working in a forensic setting could be distressing to the participants. Whilst this was not anticipated, arrangements were in place, such as sufficient time after the interview and contact numbers should the participants wish, to discuss the issues at other times.

The author of the study was a member of the professional group from which the participants were recruited. Consideration was given to this, and all the selected participants worked in the male directorate while the author worked in the women's directorate. The two directorates also have different clinical management structures.

Interviews were carried out in the participants' offices at a time convenient to them. Prior to the interview each participant was reminded of the purpose of the study, that they could withdraw at any time, and the confidentiality of the individual's data was reiterated.

The interviews took about sixty to ninety minutes, were tape-recorded and subsequently were transcribed verbatim by a person not known to the participants.

Assessing the rigour and the quality of the analysis

Independent audit

Independent audit sets out to check the validity of the reading and analysis of the participants' interviews by the researcher and the author. Having an independent researcher verifying a sample of transcripts does this. As is proposed by Smith, Jarman, and Osborn (1999), the author gave two full randomly chosen transcripts, with fully analysed information including the emergent themes and main themes, to a clinical psychologist experienced in the use of the IPA who agreed to act as an independent auditor for this research.

Respondent validity

The important process of validation of the results, referred to as "respondent validation" or "member checking" (Mays & Pope, 2000), was carried out. This involves sending to the participants the summary of the results of the analysis of their interview in written form and inviting them to comment, should they wish to do so, on the fit of the results with their experience of the interview. Individual summaries of the results were prepared for each participant. Each participant was also sent a summary of all the themes from all the participants. All the data were anonymised. This form of validation gives feedback to both the researcher and the participants about the process.

Data analysis: procedure of the IPA

The audiotapes were transcribed verbatim and analysed using the IPA (Smith, Jarman, & Osborn, 1999; Smith, Flowers, & Larkin, 2009). The transcripts were read and analysed one at a time. The analysis of each transcript was a separate and a new process even though it was the intention of the research project to search for shared themes and experiences across the group of participants. According to Smith, Jarman, and Osborn (1999), if the research explores a number of participants' transcripts they suggest two possible approaches: either using the themes list from the first interview to start with, then look for the same themes and identify new ones as they arise; or, as was done in this study, to approach the analysis of each interview anew and look for the shared themes after all the analyses had been completed.

Procedure for identifying the emergent and super-ordinate themes

The process followed the sequence suggested by Smith, Jarman, and Osborn (1999). Initially the text of the interview is read and re-read, generating exploratory comments characterised as follows:

- Descriptive comments—focusing on the content of the interview
- Linguistic comments—focusing on the use of language, on how the content is presented, looking for metaphors, hesitations, similes, etc.
- Conceptual comments—this is the more interpretative part of the analysis and is more interrogative.

The next stage of the analysis consisted of the development of emergent themes. Emergent themes are defined by Smith and colleagues as "not only the participant's original words and thoughts but also the analyst's interpretations. They reflect a synergistic process of description and interpretation" (Smith, Jarman, & Osborn, 1999, p. 92).

This stage of the analysis uses, as the material to work with, the exploratory comments obtained from the original text (rather than the original text itself) whilst "maintaining complexity, in terms of mapping the interrelationships, connections and patterns between exploratory notes" (Smith, Jarman, & Osborn, 1999, p. 92). At this stage the process becomes a reflection of both the analyst and the participant, as it is the analyst's description and interpretation of the original text. It is to some extent the researcher's judgment how the original material is interpreted. This forms the emergent themes.

The next stage consisted of drawing together the emergent themes and producing a structure to highlight the most important and interesting elements of the participants' accounts. The emergent themes can be connected in order to form meaningful clusters through a number of different patterns thus forming "super-ordinate" themes. This involved putting together emergent themes that shared conceptual elements and could be grouped together under a super-ordinate theme title/name. These super-ordinate themes were generated for each interview.

All the super-ordinate themes for each participant were collected and examined. When these were identified, extracts from the transcripts were picked out to illustrate the themes. The next stage consisted of a search for patterns and connections—exploring patterns and relationships within and between the conceptual groups, thinking about how different groups come together to help understand participants' experiences, moving from the fragments of the text to the text as a whole again.

Procedure for identifying the main themes

Following the analysis of each individual interview, each participant's super-ordinate themes were gathered, supported by emergent themes, illustrated by extracts from the interview. This process was followed for each participant. Whilst some super-ordinate themes were very similar for each participant (e.g., dichotomy), some had a slightly different, individual slant (e.g., impact; impact and its experience; impact and experience of extremes).

The individual lists of the super-ordinate themes with emergent themes were identified, maintaining the individuality of each contribution and bearing in mind the ideographic commitment of the IPA, before moving to the search for any connections between the interviews. A cluster of closely related super-ordinate themes, derived from a number of interviews, formed a main theme.

Figures 1 to 3 (below) describe the development of the themes:

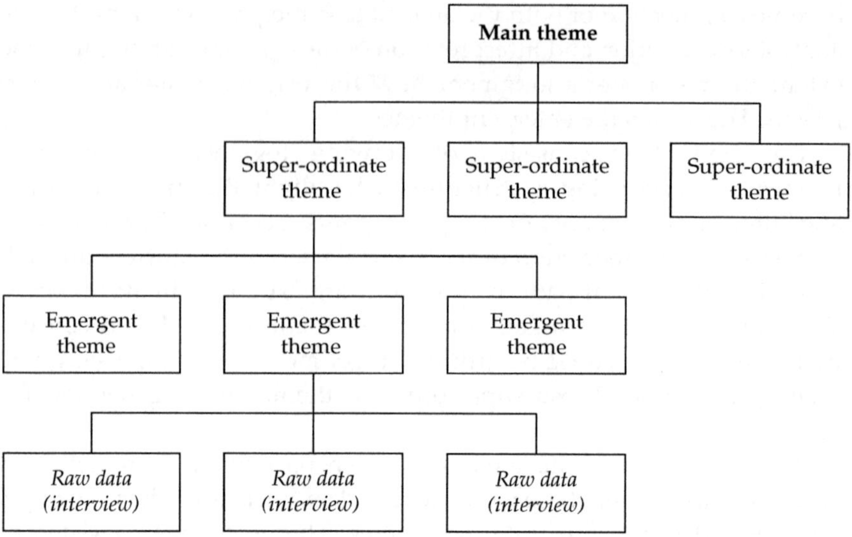

Figure 1. Development of themes—from raw data to main theme.

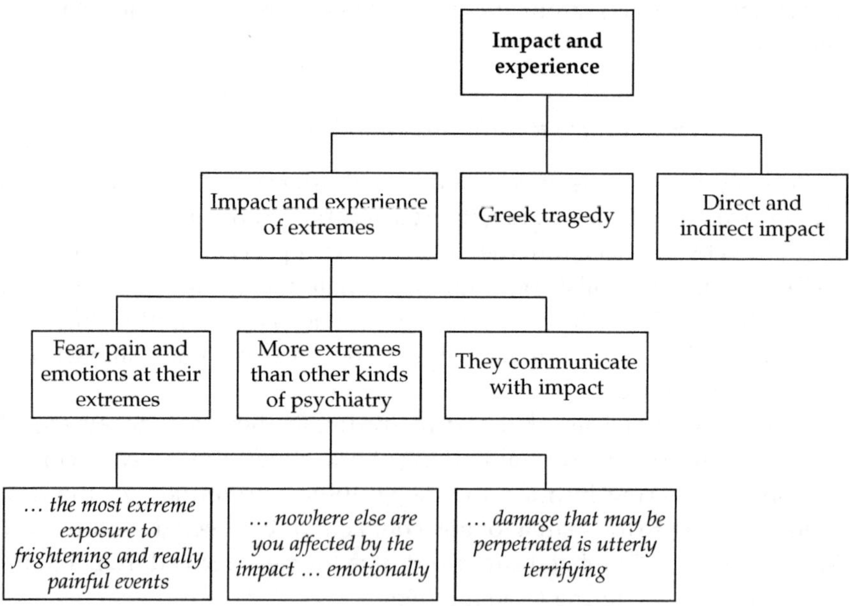

Figure 2. Example of development of a theme in cluster A, main theme 1: Impact and experience.

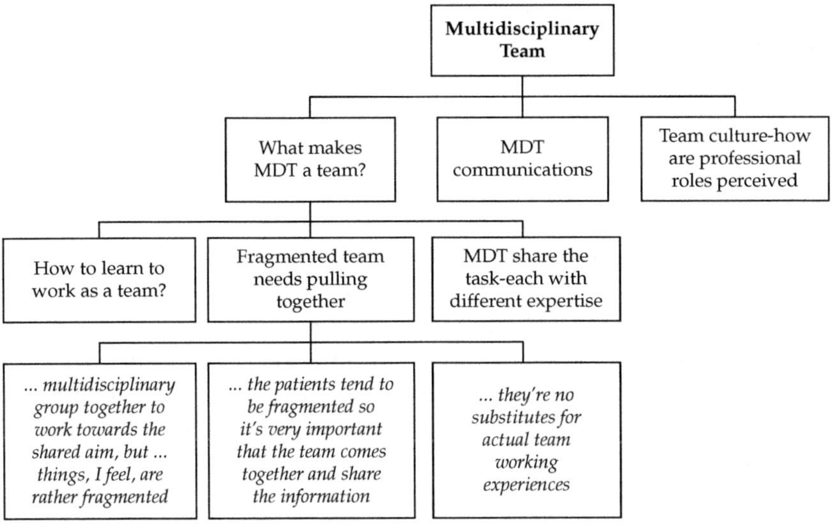

Figure 3. Example of development of a theme in cluster B, main theme 7: Multidisciplinary Team (MDT).

Thirteen such main themes were identified (see Figure 4) of which twelve were shared by more than half of the participants. These main themes were as follows: (in brackets are the number of participants who identified the theme)

- Multidisciplinary team (7)
- Interpersonal dynamics (7)
- Impact and experience (6)
- Violence and risk (6)
- Look under the surface (6)
- Dichotomy of task (5)
- Nature of the job (5)
- Professional identity (5)
- Training and preparation (5)
- Staff support (5)
- Systems issues (4)
- Communication (4).

Two participants identified the following main theme:

- Boundaries (2).

Some of the themes were strongly related to other themes, some overlapped in the participants' discussion, whilst some had only weak links to other themes.

Of the thirteen main themes identified, each consisted of varied but clearly related super-ordinate themes. These main themes reflected, not surprisingly, the sampling and the nature of the questions in the interview. The purposive sampling targeted colleagues who were familiar with the use of the ID approach; the interview explored the experience of working in multidisciplinary teams in a forensic setting.

The process of the IPA identified the presence of themes and their content. Some themes, for example "training and preparation", included various different elements from respondents, while other themes had very similar content, for example "dichotomy of task" (custodial and caring) was described by all respondents in a similar way.

The analysis of the super-ordinate and the main themes revealed that the themes gravitated into two clusters, shown in Figures 4 and 5, one with contents relating to the issues of aggression and violence (shown by a thick black line) and one that related to team-working (shown with a dotted line). Within these clusters the majority of the main themes either overlapped or were strongly linked (see Figure 5).

The additional main theme (dashed line), training and preparation, maintained an association with the two main clusters but no overlap in the emergent and the super-ordinate themes.

The first (thick black line) cluster of themes included six main themes with the content relating to aggression and violence, these were:

- Impact and experience
- Violence and risk
- Look beneath the surface
- Dichotomy of task
- Nature of job
- Boundaries.

The second (dotted line) cluster included six main themes relating to team—working, these were as follows:

- Multidisciplinary Team (MDT)
- Interpersonal Dynamics (ID)
- Staff support

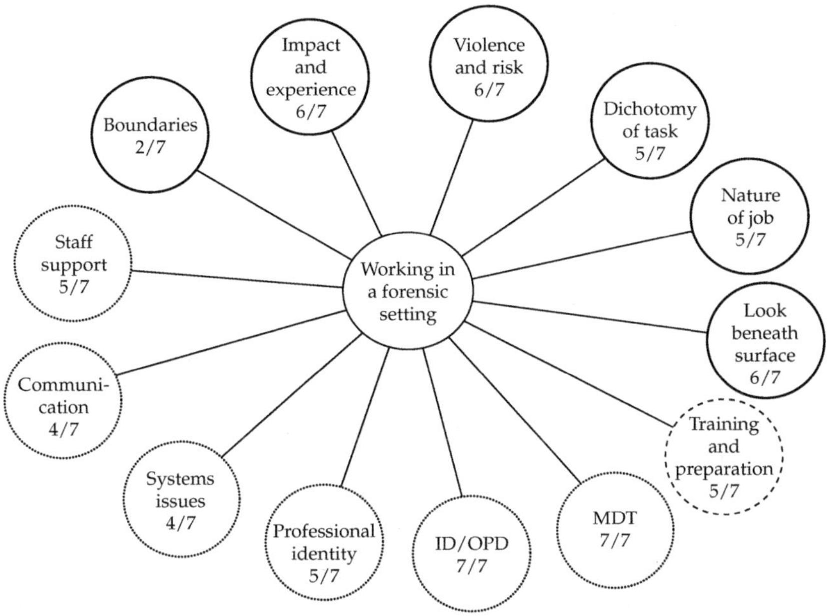

Figure 4. Main themes.

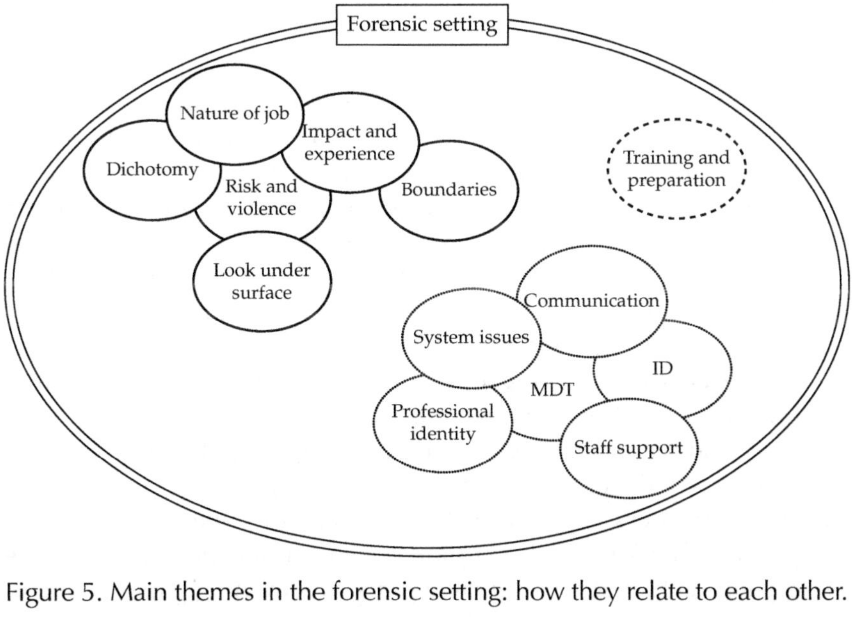

Figure 5. Main themes in the forensic setting: how they relate to each other.

- Professional identity
- Systems issues
- Communications.

The main theme that had some links to both clusters was training and preparation but it did not overlap with any other main theme and consequently belonged to neither cluster.

Discussion

The themes in the first cluster seemed to reflect more on the experiences of forensic work and related concerns and thoughts of an individual, while those in the second cluster reflected more on organisational issues faced and dealt with by a team or a group.

Training and preparation had conceptual links to both clusters but, surprisingly, was somewhat disconnected from both in the emergent and super-ordinate themes.

The study elicited and analysed the subjective experiences of working of a number of senior clinicians from a single medium secure psychiatric service. The analysis identified a number of linked themes, and from consideration of these, and from reviewing the relevant research, two main conclusions emerged;

(1) Management by the MDT and its members of the impact of violence (whether actual or potential) and of the fear generated by the interpersonal dynamics inherent in forensic work is not as effective as it needs to be. These intense feelings are often not well understood or communicated, but they are often if unknowingly acted upon by staff. In other words the countertransference permeates the staff members' experience of their work, and furthermore influences how they work. It is concluded that, for this to be addressed, there is a need for an effective mechanism to enable this impact to be managed for the individual, the team, and the service. One such mechanism is the use of Interpersonal Dynamics. ID as a systematic, methodical, and valid way to manage countertransference potentially gives all members of the team a shared understanding of these processes.
(2) MDT members experience the need for effective structures that promote thinking and communication within the team, and the organisation, and they articulate this as a training gap. In spite of

> considering themselves able and professionally competent, the participants consider from their experience that they are, nonetheless, incompletely equipped to undertake the task that is expected of them. They infer from this that they lack some unspecified, further, training.

It is a conclusion of this study that what is lacking is not training per se, but the acquisition, establishment, refinement, and use throughout the MDT of a range of processes and structures (including some existing ones) that recognise, interpret, and allow the proper management and effective communication of the impact of the transference and counter-transference from this group of patients on the service and on its staff. It is the case that training may be required to use some of these processes, but it is not the training as such, but the establishment of the right processes, and their embedding in and throughout the teams, that are necessary to address what is reported as missing in staff's readiness for the task. Existing mechanisms, such as ward rounds, reflective practice, MDT meetings, and managerial structures, do not in their current form adequately recognise, and thereby respond to, this crucial element of working with the forensic patient population.

Conclusion

This study set out to explore the staff's experience of working with forensic patients. It took place in a medium secure unit. The areas of interest were the perspectives and experiences of the participants of working as members of a MDT; their views on their core trainings and how they prepared them for their work in the forensic setting; and what organisational structures were available to carry out the job that was expected of them. In order to achieve this, seven senior members of staff were interviewed. The participants were of various core disciplines, and all contributed in different ways to the work of multidisciplinary teams.

The study identified thirteen main themes of which twelve were identified by more than half of the participants. The themes gravitated to two clusters and an outlying theme. The first cluster consisted of themes concerned with issues of aggression and violence, and the second cluster concerned themes related to team work. "Training and preparation" lay outside the two clusters but was related to both and reflected a sense of unpreparedness in the respondents, which the author concluded represented a lack of an embedded and recognised mechanism, to be used throughout the service, that would allow proper communication and management of, the clinicians' experiences. The study identified ID as a valuable tool that may be employed to address the issues identified.

References

Aiyegbusi, A., & Tuck, G. (2008). Caring amid victims and perpetrators: trauma and forensic mental health nursing. In: J. Gordon & G. Kirtchuk (Eds.), *Psychic Assaults and Frightened Clinicians* (pp. 11–26). London: Karnac.

Giorgi, A., & Giorgi, B. (2008). Phenomenology. In: J. A. Smith (Ed.), *Qualitative Psychology. A Practical Guide to Research Methods* (pp. 26–52). London: Sage Publications.

Happel, B., Pinikahana, J., & Martin, T. (2003). Stress and burnout in forensic psychiatric nursing. *Stress and Health, 19*: 63–68.

Humphreys, M. (2005). The multidisciplinary team and clinical team meetings. In: S. Wix & M. Humphreys (Eds.), *Multidisciplinary Working in Forensic Mental Health Care* (pp. 35–52). London: Elsevier.

Larkin, M., Watts, S., & Clifton, W. (2006). Giving voice and making sense in interpretative phenomenological analysis. *Qualitative Research in Psychology, 3*: 102–120.

Liberman, P. R., Hilty, D. M., Drake, R. E., & Tsang, H. W. H. (2001). Multidisciplinary roles in the 21st century: Requirements for multidisciplinary teamwork in psychiatric rehabilitation. *Psychiatric Services, 52*: 1331–1342.

Mason, T., & Carton, G. (2002). Towards a 'forensic lens' model of multidisciplinary training. *Journal of Psychiatric and Mental Health Nursing, 9*: 541–551.

Mays, N., & Pope, C. (2000). Qualitative research in healthcare: Assessing quality in qualitative research. *British Medical Journal, 320*: 50–52.

Reid, K., Flowers, P., & Larkin, M. (2005). Exploring lived experience. *Psychologist, 18*: 20–23.

Shaw, R. (2001). Why use interpretative phenomenological analysis in Health Psychology? *Health Psychology Update, 10*: 48–52.

Smith, J. A. (1995). Semi-structured interviewing and qualitative analysis. In: J. A. Smith, R. Harre, & L. Van Langehove (Eds.), *Rethinking Methods in Psychology* (pp. 9–26). London: Sage Publications.

Smith, J. A. (2004). Reflecting on the development of interpretative phenomenological analysis and its contribution to qualitative research in psychology. *Qualitative Research in Psychology, 1*: 39–54.

Smith, J. A., & Osborn, M. (2008). Interpretative Phenomenological Analysis. In: J. A. Smith (Ed.), *Qualitative Psychology* (pp. 53–80). London: Sage Publications.

Smith, J. A., Flowers, P., & Larkin, M. (2009). *Interpretative Phenomenological Analysis. Theory, Method and Research*. London: Sage Publications.

Smith, J. A., Jarman, M., & Osborn, M. (1999). Doing interpretative phenomenological analysis. In: M. Murray & K. Chamberlaine (Eds.), *Qualitative Health Psychology: Theories and Methods* (pp. 218–240). London: Sage Publications.

Willig, C. (2008). *Introducing Qualitative Research Methods in Psychology: Adventures in Theory and Method (2nd ed.)*. Maidenhead, UK: McGraw Hill/Open University Press.

Wix, S., Riordan, S., & Humphreys, M. (2005). Multidisciplinary research. In: S. Wix & M. Humphreys (Eds.), *Multidisciplinary Working in Forensic Mental Health Care* (pp. 200–213). London: Elsevier.

CHAPTER TWO

Attachment, mentalization, and the ID consultation

Gill McGauley

Introduction

Broadly speaking interpersonal interactions and relationships comprise the fora where signs and symptoms of our patients' difficulties and psychopathology are manifest. It is therefore crucial that we, as mental health professionals, are able to think about and formulate our patients' subjective experiences and the dynamics which underlie these to aid our therapeutic endeavours. One of the strengths of the Interpersonal Dynamics (ID) consultation model is that it provides clinicians and teams with a systematic way of approaching this task. The ID consultation, with its active and reactive perspectives, is centred in the subjective and relational present and recent past of the patient and the staff. This chapter first considers how the patient's distant relational past may have led to the characteristic patterns in her current interpersonal interactions and reviews the role that one particular social factor, attachment, may have in the development of adult psychopathology. The earliest experiences of attachment shape the patient's current style of interpersonal interactions and contribute to equipping the individual with an intrapsychic mental mechanism for understanding the interpersonal world: the capacity to mentalize. The second part of the chapter explores potential links between the ID consultation and attachment styles and components of mentalization in terms of the demands this approach makes on the capacity of the patient and staff to mentalize.

What determines adult psychopathology?

As a generalisation there are two views regarding which factors determine the development of psychopathology in adulthood; those who propose that the main factors are environmental and those who view biological factors, such as genetic endowment, as key. Until relatively recently the narrative explanation of mental disorder and psychopathology was that they were determined almost exclusively by environmental and social factors, particularly the family system (Bowlby, 1951; Brown & Harris, 1978; Rutter, 2005a, 2005b; Winnicott, 1963). The dominant model of environmental factors has been severely challenged in the last thirty years by the rapid growth of human genetic research and the mapping of the human genome (McGuffin, Riley, & Plomin, 2001; Plomin & Bergeman, 1991; Rutter, Silberg, O'Connor, & Simonoff, 1999). Some researchers postulate that the pendulum has swung too far and that the ascendancy of genomics has eclipsed the contribution of environmental, particularly social, determinants of childhood and adult psychopathology (Fonagy, 2003a; Kendler, 2005).

The environmental contribution to psychiatric disorder and the gene–environment interaction

Many research studies have shown substantial and significant associations between a wide range of environmental risk factors and psychopathological outcomes (Rutter, 1971; Rutter, 2005b; Rutter, Kreppner, & O'Connor, 2001). The favoured interpretation of these associations was that risky environmental mechanisms were causal in the development of mental disorder, and most childhood and adult psychopathology were seen as the sequelae of environmental risk factors; parental influences were thought to be particularly important. Contemporary approaches conceptualise psychopathology in a framework that includes social as well as genetic determinants (Kandel, 1998). Development involves gene–environment interactions. Genes may moderate social risk factors; however, social factors may predispose to the development of psychopathology as they can both give rise to adverse events as well as increasing the individual's vulnerability to such events (Harris, Brown, & Bifulco, 1986). One pathway suggests that the social environment triggers genetic susceptibility; for example, in the Dunedin cohort both antisocial behaviour in males and depression in males and females have been linked to gene variants but only for individuals exposed to stressful early life environments (Caspi et al., 2002–2004).

The role of attachment in the development of psychopathology

The nature of the main environmental experiences that carry risk are seen as social and, to a greater or lesser extent, involve the attachment system. Risk derived from situations where social and interpersonal relationships have not been formed (O'Connor et al., 2003; Rutter, Kreppner, & O'Connor, 2001; Rutter, 2004); where the security of these relationships has been disrupted by neglect or abuse (Cicchetti, 2004); or where the quality of the adult-child interaction has been sub-optimal (Rutter, 2005a, 2005b).

There is wide variation in the individual's response to social risk factors; some individuals decompensate and develop a mental disorder, some emerge unaffected and some appear strengthened. This heterogeneity of response is poorly understood (Rutter, 2005a; 2005b) but suggests that intrapsychic variables have a contribution. Importantly, whether an environmental factor triggers a genetic predisposition to psychopathology may depend, not only on the factor itself, but on the way the individual *experiences* the environmental factor. In other words the subjective experience of the environment acts as a filter in the mediation of the genotype to the phenotype. Attachment has been proposed as one such intrapsychic filter (Fonagy, 2003a).

There is considerable research evidence linking attachment and its disruption to both abnormal developmental trajectories and the development of poor mental health and psychopathology (DeKlyen & Greenberg, 2008; Lyons-Ruth, Alpern, & Repacholi, 1993; Sroufe, 2005). In summary:

- Abnormal social attachments characterise virtually every form of psychopathology (Insel & Winslow, 2004).
- The formation of adequate early social and interpersonal relationships is one of the key environmental determinants of mental health.

- Environmental factors that severely restrict the development of attachment relationships, as in institutional or other extremely deprived rearing environments, affect mental health (O'Connor, 2006).
- Severe disruptions in or threats to the security of relationships which result from abuse, neglect, and rejection are risk factors for the development of psychopathology (Cicchetti & Toth, 1995).

Attachment theory—from observation to representation

What is attachment theory, and how do attachment and early developmental experiences shape an individual's social and interpersonal world?

Attachment theory is a body of knowledge concerned with the emotional bonds and affective interactions between human beings and the psychological difficulties and psychopathological consequences which arise when these processes go awry (Bowlby, 1977). In other words, it is about how we relate to those to whom we are closest.

In classical attachment theory, as developed by John Bowlby and Mary Ainsworth (Ainsworth, Blehar, Waters, & Wall, 1978; Bowlby, 1969, 1973, 1977, 1980, 1988), the attachment bond between the baby and its primary caregiver (most often the mother) was necessary for the baby's protection and security. Bowlby drew on evidence from ethological studies to question the, at the time, widely accepted psychoanalytic secondary-drive theory that the baby's relationship with the mother arises because she feeds the baby (Freud, 1957). Lorenz (1935) had observed that infant geese become attached to parents and objects that did not feed them and Harlow (1958), in his eloquent study of infant rhesus monkeys, concluded that under stress the infant monkeys preferred the cloth covered "mother" that provided comfort through contact rather than the wire-mesh "mother" that provided food. Ainsworth's (1967) pioneering systematic observational work established that babies also established attachments to people who did not feed them (Cassidy, 2008).

In summary, Bowlby proposed that the attachment bond developed as an evolutionary mechanism to promote the security and survival of the infant. Bowlby postulated that this bond forms during the first year of life and continues as part of the normal repertoire of child and adult behaviour. Attachment behaviour is most obvious when there is a threat, real or perceived, to this bond. In these situations, the child, distressed on the withdrawal of the attachment figure, shows a strong tendency to seek proximity with the attachment figure, especially when in pain or frightened. Disruption or the threat of disruption of these bonds through separation, bereavement, deprivation, neglect, or abuse stimulates painful affective states and in some cases leads to psychopathology. In Bowlby and Ainsworth's view, a child uses the attachment figure as a "secure base" from which to explore the world. Through this process the child constructs mental representations or internal working models (Bowlby, 1973) of their attachment figures, of himself and the relationships between these representations. As well as the evolutionary advantage that a strong affectional bond to a caregiver bestows on a vulnerable infant, these internal working models encode the meaning of attachment experience which then guides expectations and behaviour (Bowlby, 1973; Steele 2003). For example, if the attachment figure has been sensitive to the infant's needs the child is likely to develop an internal working model of the self as valued. If, however, the parent has been rejecting the child is likely to construct an internal model of the self as unworthy or incompetent (Bretherton, 1995). These internal working models not only integrate past experiences but also regulate the child's behaviour with attachment figures and come to organise and predict behaviour in future attachment relationships (Bretherton & Munholland, 1999).

The construct of internal working models was an extremely important development as it allowed attachment theory to make its own developmental leap, for it meant that attachment research could move from the observational level, where behaviours were observed, counted and coded, to the representational level of internal mental states. Furthermore internal working models provided a mechanism for both linking the sequelae of adverse early attachment experiences to the development of psychopathology and for understanding how early attachment experiences can be replayed in interpersonal relationships across the lifespan.

Consequently, the contribution of attachment to development has now extended beyond its classic role in ensuring the survival of the infant through establishing attachment relationships to equipping the person with an intrapsychic mechanism which acts to process experience and allows the person to represent mental states of the self and other and understand the interpersonal world (Fonagy, 2003a; Steele, 2003). In summary attachment:

- Allows for the development of a representational system
- The representational system allows for the processing of experience

- The way in which experience is processed can moderate the expression of genotypical and environmental determinants of adult psychopathology.

Contemporary interest in attachment has grown precisely because early attachment experiences provide the tools that the mind uses to develop capacities such as affect and stress regulation and the capacity to mentalize; capacities that bestow an evolutionary advantage (Luyten, Fonagy, Lowyck, & Vermote, 2012).

ID, attachment, personality development, and its pathology

The ID consultation offers clinicians and teams a way of developing a shared understanding of the characteristic interpersonal interactions of their patients. It draws heavily on Benjamin's Structural Analysis of Social Behaviour (SASB), a method of describing and analysing interpersonal interactions (Benjamin, 1996). Benjamin's approach shares some assumptions with attachment theory, namely, that individuals have an inborn need to form attachments; that these attachments are represented mentally and that early ways of being related to and the representations that subsequently develop guide future interpersonal interactions. However, to what extent do early developmental experiences shape our ability to regulate our interpersonal interactions and contribute to the development of psychopathology?

Much of the early attachment research studies looked at attachment in low-risk, non-clinical populations. In the last two decades attachment research has broadened to include clinical and other high-risk groups such as those facing social adversity (poverty or social exclusion); those with mental health and substance misuse disorders or those who have offended or are violent. The following review concentrates on studies in clinical and high-risk groups and explores the relationship between the child's attachment status and the development of psychopathology; evidence is examined as to whether specific attachment states of mind are associated with particular psychiatric disorders and psychopathologies. It concentrates on studies that have assessed attachment in children using the Strange Situation Procedure (SSP) (Ainsworth, Blehar, Waters, & Wall, 1978) and the Adult Attachment Interview (AAI) for adults (George, Kaplan, & Main, 1996; Main, Goldwyn, & Hesse, 2003). The development of these first assessment tools provided a way of systematically classifying infant attachment and attachment states of mind in adults. Although several other assessment tools have been developed for use in other populations (Bifulco, Moran, Ball, & Bernazzani, 2002; Crittenden, 2000), the SSP and AAI have been used in the majority of studies and are briefly outlined here.

In the SSP, children, upon reunion with their primary attachment figure, react in one of three ways. Infants who actively seek contact with their caregiver on reunion, communicate their feelings of stress and distress openly and then readily return to exploratory play are classified as secure in their attachment to that caregiver. Children who do not appear distressed and ignore or avoid their caregiver on reunion (although, like secure children, they are physiologically aroused during the separation) are classified as insecure—avoidant. Children who combine strong proximity seeking with resistance to contact, or who remain unsoothable without being able to return to explore and play, are classified as insecure—ambivalent attached. When faced with having to modulate between attachment and exploration, ambivalent infants maximise attachment behaviours, whereas avoidant infants minimise or deactivate attachment behaviours and conceal their distress. Secure infants achieve a balance between activating attachment behaviours on reunion and subsequently returning to explorative play (van IJzendoorn & Bakermans-Kranenburg, 1997). Main and Solomon (1989) identified a fourth category, that of disorganised/disorientated behaviour, during the SSP. These children showed contradictory or undirected behaviour such as freezing or stereotypic movements or signs of apprehension regarding the parent. Further research showed that the parents of these children were in a state of unresolved mourning in relation to earlier losses or traumas (Main & Hesse, 1990) or had abused or neglected their children (Carlson, Cicchetti, Barnett, & Braunwald, 1989).

Broadly speaking an individual is classified as secure on the AAI if they value attachment relationships and are able to describe them objectively, irrespective of whether these experiences were negative or positive. Secure individuals have coherent attachment narratives where they are able to think about their attachment figures and their own experiences in a balanced way. Insecurely attached individuals who are "dismissing" of attachment are dismissing, devaluing or cut-off from attachment relationships and experiences. Insecurely attached "preoccupied" individuals are confused, un-objective, and preoccupied with past attachment relationships and experiences. Superimposed upon these categories is the unresolved/disorganised category with respect to loss or trauma in relation to an attachment figure (Main & Solomon, 1989). These individuals show a localised lack of coherency in their thinking around loss and trauma (Main & Hesse, 1992) signaling a breakdown in internal mental mechanisms for coping with stress. However, in other areas of the AAI, an unresolved individual may be coherent. A fourth category, cannot classify, was introduced into the coding system in 1994 (Hesse, 1996). Placement in this category indicates that the individual has a disorganised state of mind with respect to attachment and cannot be classified as being dismissing, preoccupied, or secure. In other words, these individuals have no overarching attachment strategy but employ two disparate and opposing strategies.

Infant, childhood, and adolescent attachment and psychopathology in high-risk populations

In high-risk groups the parental factors shown to increase the risk of children developing psychopathology include parental psychopathology, lower levels of parental support, teenage parenting and substance abuse (Kobak, Cassidy, Lyons-Ruth, & Ziv, 2006). The Minnesota Parent–Child Project (Sroufe, 2005), a major longitudinal study with follow-up into late adolescence, showed that children with insecure attachment patterns who were raised in high-risk environments were more likely to have poor peer relations, exhibit depressive symptoms and show more symptoms of aggression and maladjustment than their securely attached counterparts. Securely attached children, on the other hand, exhibit lower levels of externalising behaviours such as aggression, delinquency, and hyperactivity (Davies, Cummings, & Winter, 2004) and internalising symptoms (depression and anxiety) and behaviours (self-harm) in middle childhood (Muris, Mayer, & Meesters, 2000). A number of studies have suggested that insecure disorganised/disorientated infants, who lack a consistent strategy for organising their responses when their attachment system is stressed, were particularly at risk of developing problem behaviours, demonstrating peer aggression (Lyons-Ruth, Alpern, & Repacholi, 1993) and experiencing dissociative symptoms in adolescence (Carlson, 1998).

However, these studies do not yield clear-cut results (Munson, McMahon, & Spieker, 2001) and drawing firm conclusions has been hampered by the small number of studies, many of which measured different symptoms and used differing methods of assessing attachment. As a broad conclusion it appears that children who form a secure attachment to their mothers are less likely to experience clinical symptoms in middle childhood, while insecure attachment is viewed as a risk factor for the development of some forms of psychopathology. Furthermore, attachment insecurity seems to be an important but non-specific factor which increases the risk of a range of childhood psychopathology (DeKlyen & Greenberg, 2008). In particular disorganised/disorientated attachment is seen as a particular vulnerability factor which increases the likelihood of children developing psychopathology and adaption problems (Sroufe, Carlson, Levy, & Egeland, 1999).

As a general statement secure attachment is associated with healthy functioning in adolescents while insecure attachment has been linked to psychopathology (Allen, Hauser, & Borman-Spurrell, 1996; Muris & Meesters, 2002). Studies suggest that preoccupied attachment states of mind predispose adolescents to developing internalising symptoms while those with dismissing states of mind were more likely to develop externalising symptoms. However, this is not a consistent pattern.

Adult attachment and psychopathology in high-risk populations

Attachment studies in adults have mainly used a cross-sectional design and examined whether specific types of attachment insecurity are associated with particular psychiatric disorders. Studies examining attachment classifications in individuals with depressive disorders and in individuals with eating disorders have yielded an inconsistent picture. Depression and eating disorders are reported as being associated with both preoccupied attachment (Cole-Detke & Kobak, 1996; Fonagy et al., 1996) and dismissing classifications (Cole-Detke & Kobak 1996; Patrick, Hobson, Castle, Howard, & Maughan, 1994; Ward et al., 2001). Studies of individuals with a diagnosis of anxiety disorder report an over-representation of both preoccupied and unresolved states of mind (Manassis, Bradley, Goldberg, Hood, & Swinson, 1994; Fonagy et al., 1996), although the latter finding was not replicated (Van Emmichoven, van IJzendoorn, de Ruiter, & Brosschot, 2003).

The relationship between attachment states of mind in schizophrenia is more consistent. All studies report that the majority of individuals were dismissing with respect to attachment (Dozier, Cue, & Barnett, 1994) with high rates of unresolved states of mind (Tyrrell, Dozier, Teague, & Fallot, 1999). The authors warn against concluding that the individuals' attachment state of mind predated their schizophrenic illness. They point out that the symptoms of schizophrenia, such as thought disorder which leads to lapses in the monitoring of reasoning and discourse, may have led to high numbers of individuals being classified as unresolved. Likewise the negative symptoms of schizophrenia may have resulted in individuals being classified as dismissing. In other words, it is unclear whether the symptoms of mental illness have disrupted the patient's attachment system or whether the AAI coding system is responding to the patient's symptoms.

Several studies have looked at the association between attachment states of mind in individuals with a diagnosis of personality disorder (PD), particularly Borderline Personality Disorder (BPD) and Antisocial Personality Disorder (ASPD) (Barone, 2003; Fonagy et al., 1996; Patrick, Hobson, Castle, Howard, & Maughan, 1994). The results consistently report that the majority of individuals with a diagnosis of BPD had preoccupied states of mind. When unresolved status was coded, eighty-nine per cent (Fonagy et al., 1996) and seventy-five per cent (Patrick, Hobson, Castle, Howard, & Maughan, 1994) of patients were classified as unresolved.

Adult attachment in forensic and violent populations

The literature has taken three approaches to investigating attachment in high-risk violent populations where violence has been directed externally as opposed to self-directed violence: (1) studies of attachment in individuals who have a psychiatric diagnosis but who have also offended violently (Frodi, Derenevik, Sepa, Philipson, & Bragesjo, 2001; Levinson & Fonagy, 2004; van IJzendoorn et al., 1997; (2) studies of attachment in inter-familial violence such as in abusive parents (Adshead & Bluglass, 2005; Crittenden, Partridge, & Claussen, 1991) where the individuals may or may not have a psychiatric disorder and in non-incarcerated men who have committed domestic/marital violence but who do not have a diagnosed psychiatric disorder (Babcock, Jacobson, Gottman, & Yerington, 2000; Holtzworth-Munroe,

Stuart, & Hutchinson, 1997); and (3) studies which have assessed attachment status in individuals who have a psychiatric diagnosis which is associated with later violence, such as conduct disordered adolescents (Allen, Hauser, & Borman-Spurrell, 1996; Rosenstein & Horowitz, 1996).

In the first group all of these studies reported an over-representation of individuals with dismissing attachment states of mind. These states of mind were statistically more likely in the violent prisoners compared to a matched non-violent group of patients with a personality disorder (Levinson & Fonagy, 2004). There was also a high level of individuals with a cannot classify attachment classification indicating a more chaotic attachment system.

In the second group of studies insecure attachments were over-represented in the study groups; however, both dismissing and preoccupied insecure attachments styles were over-represented. Domestically violent men were more likely to have an insecure attachment status, and dismissing attachment organisation was associated with higher antisocial scores (Babcock, Jacobson, Gottman, & Yerington, 2000). In mothers who have abused their children an over-representation of both dismissing and preoccupied attachment states of mind have been described (Adshead & Bluglass, 2005); Crittenden, Partridge, & Claussen, 1991).

When considering conduct disorder, which can lead developmentally to violent offending, the findings remained relatively consistent with those adolescents who had dismissing attachment states of mind being more likely to have a conduct disorder. In the only longitudinal attachment study, insecure attachment organisation at the age of twenty-five was linked to self-reported criminal behaviour as well as hard drug use ten years later (Allen, Hauser, & Borman-Spurrell, 1996). The cannot classify subgroup reported the most criminal behaviour while the dismissing and unresolved individuals had higher levels of criminal behaviour compared with the preoccupied and securely attached individuals.

In summary there are few empirical studies which have examined attachment and violence and even fewer which have looked at violence in individuals with a psychiatric disorder. The literature is further complicated by studies which use samples of individuals who both have a psychiatric disorder but who are also violent, so it is not possible to ascertain whether insecure attachment is associated with the psychiatric disorder, the violent behaviour or both.

In conclusion, although the last decade has seen an expansion of attachment research to include psychiatric groups, examination of the empirical literature to investigate whether particular attachment classifications are associated with specific psychopathologies or psychiatric disorders in adulthood has often lacked a systematic approach; notable exceptions are the meta-analyses and review conducted by Bakermans-Kranenburg and van IJzendoorn (Bakermans-Kranenburg & van IJzendoorn, 2009; van IJzendoorn & Bakermans-Kranenburg, 1996) and Kobak and colleagues' review (Kobak, Cassidy, Lyons-Ruth, & Ziv, 2006). Overall these studies indicated that individuals with psychiatric diagnoses showed more insecure and unresolved attachment representations than non-clinical groups. Disorders with an internalising dimension (e.g., borderline personality disorder) were associated with more preoccupied and unresolved attachments.

However, both dismissing and preoccupied attachments were over-represented in externalising disorders such as antisocial personality disorder (ASPD). Although it is reasonable to conclude that there is an association between insecure attachment status and psychopathology, the data are not yet robust enough to conclude whether insecure attachment status constitutes a general risk factor for mental health or whether specific types of attachment insecurity are associated with particular psychiatric disorders.

Mentalization—the legacy of attachment

The capacity to mentalize, that is, to ascribe meaning to human behaviour which ultimately shapes our understanding of others and ourselves, develops within early secure attachment relationships where we experience our internal states being understood by another mind (Fonagy, 2003b; Koren-Karie, Oppenheim, Dolev, Sher, & Etzion-Carasso, 2002). As mentioned above, the contribution of attachment to personality development therefore extends beyond its role in ensuring infant survival and generating internal working models to equipping the person with an intrapsychic mental mechanism: the capacity to mentalize. Mentalization allows the individual to process experience and to represent mental states of the self and other (Fonagy, 2003a, 2003b; Steele, 2003). It includes the ability to distinguish one's own mental states from those of others and to be able to understand and interpret the actions and behaviour of oneself and others as meaningful and based on intentional mental states (Allen, 2008). Findings from empirical studies show that securely attached children outperform insecure children on mentalizing tasks (de Rosnay & Harris, 2002). However the development of healthy mentalizing is thought to depend on more than just a secure attachment relationship with caregivers. The emotional availability of the caretaker and the degree to which attachment figures adequately mirror the infant's subjective experience are also important. In particular, the capacity of the attachment figure to relate to the child as an individual with her own mental states is seen as crucially important for the development of mentalization (Fonagy, Luyten, & Strathearn, 2011).

So what does poor mentalizing look like? There are many variations, but at its core there is a failure in the patients' narrative to describe experience in terms of mental states, that is, in terms of thoughts, feelings, or intentions. Instead individuals might talk about external social factors such as their environment or the physical characteristics of their attachment figures and associates. Their thoughts and feelings about others are also held with certainty. They are sure that they know what the other is feeling and thinking, and this certainty bars them from being able to consider any other perspective. Denial of involvement in a problem and a sense of agency are also characteristically lacking as there is an unwillingness to look at one's own and others' intentions. When an already fragile mentalizing system is stressed either by high affect arousal or activation of the attachment system prementalizing and primitive modes of experiencing the self and others emerge. For example in pretend mode the speaker's narrative is cut off from any meaningful link to his internal experience and at the extreme may have a dissociative quality. In an attempt to find a connection to his feelings the patient may talk extensively but the connection often seems random or confusing to the listener and further exploration fails to clarity. For example, a patient who is separated from her children begins to talk about how she misses them but her narrative lacks emotion and she quickly jumps to talk about how the trees she can see through the window are like those in the woods she used to walk in (ten years ago) and provides the listener with a detailed description of these walks as if she was talking about the recent past. In psychic equivalence mode the individual's internal experience is real and there is no room for doubt. If the individual "thinks" that the world is a certain way then it is; internal and external reality are equivalent. The patient will therefore know what is on another person's mind or why they did what they did. In a teleological mode of prementalizing functioning the individual equates mental states with observable behaviour as the only way the speaker can work out the minds of others is by their actions: "as you were late for our meeting you think I am worthless." These non-mentalizing modes of experiencing can severely disrupt and disorganise interpersonal relationships (Fonagy, Bateman, & Luyten, 2012).

Mentalizing in forensic and violent populations

The above descriptors capture many of the characteristic ways forensic and offender patients think, feel, experience, and react in interpersonal interactions. Several studies confirm that offenders in prison or in secure forensic institutions are more likely to have experienced separations, abuse, and neglect from their early caregivers compared to individuals in the general population (Coid, 1992; Pert, Ferriter, & Saul, 2004) and consequently in adulthood have insecure attachment states of mind. They have either not had the continuity of early attachment relationships, in which the child can learn about mental states, or their experience of maltreatment from attachment figures has turned the child's mind away from taking the perspective of the other as to do so would expose the child to the hostility in the abuser's mind which is directed towards her (Cicchetti, 2004; O'Connor, 2006). Early abuse, neglect, and violence impact on the child's developing capacity for emotional regulation and mentalizing. Fonagy and colleagues (Fonagy, 2003b; Levinson & Fonagy, 2004), in their developmental model of violence, suggest that the early determinants of insecure attachment states of mind, such as adverse environments (including disrupted or trauma infused attachment experiences) coupled with gene–environment interactions lead to a disavowal of attachment experiences and of the capacity to mentalize. Conversely it is known that the formation of healthy attachment relationships acts as a protective factor and may divert the child away from a pathway of violence and behavioural disturbance as, through such relationships, the child can learn about the other as another human being (Fonagy, 2003b; O'Connor, Marvin, Rutter, Olrick, & Britner, 2003; Rutter, Kreppner, & O'Connor, 2001). Trauma is a particular threat to the developing capacity to mentalize. In their model Allen, Lemma, and Fonagy (2012) emphasise the dual liability that stems from traumatic childhood attachments which not only stimulate extreme distress but also impair the child's capacity to regulate emotional distress, partly through compromising the development of mentalizing. These individuals show deficits in empathy and struggle to differential their own mental state from that of others. In the face of subsequent trauma mentalizing breaks down.

The capacity to mentalize is thought to be a crucial inhibitory factor for interpersonal violence, and it is hypothesised that a deficit in mentalizing (Fonagy et al., 1997) is a critical mediating mechanism between insecure states of mind and violent behaviour as it might remove an inhibitory barrier to violence (Levinson & Fonagy, 2004). This mechanism may be particularly active in individuals with antisocial personality disorder (ASPD), many of whom have insecure-dismissing attachment states of mind in which they devalue and denigrate attachment relationships. McGauley, Yakeley, Williams & Bateman (2011) and Yakeley (2014) describe how these individuals, because of their compromised capacity to mentalize, cannot tolerate negative emotions and impulses such as anger, hatred, and a wish to hurt others; they become highly aroused and overwhelmed with negative affects. Additionally people with ASPD are sensitive to both real and perceived threats to their self-worth. Poor mentalizing means that they can frequently misread and misperceive the minds and actions of others, "seeing" slights, insults, and markers of disrespect all too easily. The feelings of shame and humiliation generated are unbearable, and poor mentalization means that these cannot be processed and contained by normal mental representational mechanisms; they are experienced concretely as feelings or sensations that need to be expelled through violence. Just as individuals with ASPD cannot contain their self-states when aroused, they fail to accurately mentalize the mind of the other which further lowers their threshold for aggression. If an individual is unable to see the other as having mental states different from himself, normal inhibitory mechanisms for violence are reduced as the soon-to-be-aggressor is unable to empathise or appreciate another person's suffering. Indeed the aggressor may so misidentify the mental state of the other as to be convinced that his victim is as angry and aroused as he is and, consequently, feel under threat and attack.

The proposed pathway linking dismissing attachment states of mind, mentalization and violent behaviour is supported by some empirical research. Mentalization can be assessed by rating AAI transcripts for reflective function (RF) which assesses the individual's capacity to understand and interpret their own and others' behaviour in terms of underlying mental states (Fonagy, Steele, Steele, Moran, & Higgitt, 1991). Levinson and Fonagy (Levinson & Fonagy, 2004) report poorer mentalization, as assessed by rf, in a violent group of prisoners whose offences were of interpersonal violence compared with prisoners who had committed non-violent offences. They propose that the violent act may occur when a person with poor mentalization cannot manage internal feeling states and therefore resorts to physical action against the other.

Although in general mentalizing is seen as a stable trait, our capacity to mentalize is influenced to a certain extent by the context, especially the context of attachment relationships. States of emotional arousal disrupt and decrease our capacity to mentalize (Luyten, Fonagy, Lowyck, & Vermote, 2012). One has only to think about what one has said in the heat of a blazing argument to a loved one and how easily we can resort to concrete thinking and non-mentalizing generalisations: "You never help me … you always criticise me."

In summary, mentalizing allows for the processing of experience and is an essential human capacity underpinning our interpersonal relations as it provides us with a capacity to think about our own attachment relationships, mental state, and the mental states of others. It has been postulated that the capacity to mentalize is a critical mediating mechanism between dismissing derogating attachment states of mind and some types of interpersonal violence. Individuals with an impaired capacity to mentalize, whether this is a context dependent failure of mentalization or a pervasive trait deficit, are more likely to be violent.

The ID consultation, attachment, and mentalization

The first part of this chapter describes the contribution that attachment makes to the development of psychopathology and in determining the colouration of the patients' social world through their interpersonal interactions. The early lives of the majority of forensic patients have been blighted by adverse attachment experiences, leaving them in adult life with disorganised and insecure ways of mentally representing attachment experiences which drive their interpersonal interactions. These mental representations are replayed within their interactions with staff and other patients at individual, team, and institutional levels and can manifest in many shades of behaviour including aggressive, dismissive, clinging, seductive, and many more styles.

One of the strengths of the ID consultation model is that it provides clinicians and teams with a systematic way of approaching the task of describing and thinking about our patients' interpersonal interactions. The ID consultation helps us look at the current legacy of attachment experiences in the area of interpersonal interactions; however, it does not claim to offer any causal mechanism for the underlying developmental processes. How then might attachment relate to the ID consultation? Perhaps the easiest way of summarising this is that attachment classifications, according to the AAI, map loosely to some of the relationship characteristics and items on both the active and reactive planes of the interpersonal circle. Through the process of administering the ID consultation, tracers of attachment styles will emerge mainly through the interpersonal perspective that relates to the patient's experience of herself (perspective B). Overall the ID clusters and items seem to relate more to insecure-dismissing rather than insecure-preoccupied attachment states of mind. For example, "allowing independence" (when the patient believes that he "needs no-one") maps loosely to the claim for independence and self-sufficiency which characterises dismissing attachment where the effect of attachment is limited and deactivated within current relationships. The controlling, blaming, and destroying clusters tap into the devaluing and derogating of attachment that characterises individuals who have highly dismissive states of mind. In these states of mind attachment figures are treated as less than human, for example, "I can force people to do whatever I want"; "I need to teach my girlfriend a lesson"; "You are dead to me". It is unsurprising that there is only a loose coupling between ID clusters and attachment categories as the tools are designed to look at differing constructs and are administered and rated differently. During an ID consultation, specific items are decided upon largely by the staff's observations of the patient's interactions and their effects on others, including the observer; whereas classifying attachment states of mind, as assessed by the AAI, rely heavily on a discourse analysis of the patient's narrative. In other words it is not only what patients say but how they describe their experiences and attachment figures that allow us to access their attachment state of mind.

The ID consultation offers clinicians a framework for describing and thinking about the interpersonal interactions of their patients within the context of the multidisciplinary team and, at its core, encourages and supports clinicians and professionals to mentalize about the minds and actions of their patients. Mentalization is a multidimensional construct which, according to Fonagy and colleagues, comprises four components (see Fonagy, Bateman, & Luyten, 2012 for a full description of these facets) each of which is linked to distinct underlying neural systems established through neuro-imaging studies of social cognition. Two of these components may be particularly stimulated when teams undertake an ID consultation on their patients; the dimension of automatic (implicit)—controlled (explicit) mentalization and that of internally focused—externally focused mentalization.

Most of the time when we interact with each other spontaneously, mentalizing happens automatically. We are unaware that we are interpreting other people's feelings and intentions and just respond to them reciprocally by making reasonable assumptions about their motives. This implicit or automatic mentalizing is the modus operandi of most professional-patient interactions. It is only when the other person departs from the expected response that automatic mentalization moves into controlled or explicit mentalization. We are often aware of this switch as we can feel surprised, curious or perplexed by the response of the other. Controlled mentalization needs our awareness and reflection and requires effort. One of the key functions of the ID consultation is that it requires staff to explicitly mentalize about both their patient's mental experience and the impact of that experience upon themselves.

The second polarity of mentalization that underpins the ID consultation is that of internally focused—externally focused mentalization. The links between this facet and the various perspectives of the ID consultation are outlined in Table 1. Internally focused mentalization refers to mental processes that focus on one's own (self-directed) or another's (other-directed) internal experiences (thoughts, feelings, and impulses), and it is this end of the continuum that the ID consultation stimulates. Externally focused mentalizing relies on physical and visible features of one's own or another's actions; for example, a patient who relies on external mentalization may assume that his primary nurse is angry with him as the nurse did not instantly greet him on coming onto the unit. The ID consultation demands that the multidisciplinary team focus on internal mental states from two perspectives; firstly, the staff team thinking about the internal mental states of the patient, that is, other directed; and secondly, asking the staff to focus on their own internal mental experiences about the patient, that is, self-directed. The ID consultation allows for the possibility of drawing on another facet of mentalization if a team member conducts a consultation with the patient to seek the

Table 1. ID consultation perspectives and the components of mentalization.

ID consultation perspective	*Component of mentalization which ID consultation draws on in the staff*	*Component of mentalization ID consultation draws on in the patient (if ID consultation interview undertaken directly with the patient)*
Perspective A: The patient repeatedly experiences others as … (focus is on the other—active)	Internal–external component: **Internally** focused mentalization but **other**–directed as asking the staff to focus on the internal mental states of the patient, that is, his thoughts and feelings. Does not pull on externally focused mentalization as staff need to move beyond inferring the patient's mental experience based on the patient's external actions and behaviour.	Self–**other** component of mentalization as assessing the extent to which the patient can accurately mentalise the minds of **others** in terms of thoughts, feelings, impulses.
Perspective B: The patient repeatedly experiences herself as … (focus is on the self–reactive)	Internal–external component: **Internally** focused but **other**–directed as asking the staff to focus on the internal mental states of the patient, that is, their thoughts and feelings. Not externally focused mentalization as staff need to move beyond inferring the patient's mental experience based on the patient's external actions and behaviour.	**Self**–other component of mentalization as assessing the extent to which the patient can accurately mentalise her **own** mind in terms of thoughts, feelings, impulses.

(*Continued*)

Table 1. Continued.

ID consultation perspective	*Component of mentalization which ID consultation draws on in the staff*	*Component of mentalization ID consultation draws on in the patient (if ID consultation interview undertaken directly with the patient)*
Perspective C: Others; the staff repeatedly experience the patient as … (focus is on the self–active)	Internal–external component: **Internally** focused mentalization but **self**–directed as asking the staff to focus on their own internal mental state, that is, their own thoughts and feelings **about** the patient.	
Perspective D: Others; the staff repeatedly experience themselves in their interactions as … (focus is on the self–reactive)	Internal–external component but **self**–directed. Asking the staff to focus on their own internal mental state **about** the patient but also on the extent to which these underpin their reactions and behaviour towards the patient.	

patient's perspective directly. In this situation the team member could gain a state dependent snap shot of the extent to which the patient can accurately mentalize her own mind and the minds of others in terms of thoughts, feelings, and impulses.

Conclusions

A disrupted attachment system, consequent on adverse attachment experiences, is just one of many factors which contribute to the development of psychopathology and poor interpersonal relationships in adulthood. However, attachment does make a specific contribution as it equips the individual with an intrapsychic mental mechanism for understanding the interpersonal world: the capacity to understand minds—to mentalize. The ID consultation offers clinicians and teams a way to systematise their thinking about their patients' subjective experience of their interpersonal behaviours and ways of relating. The ID consultation can reveal the fixed and rigid ways in which the patient "time and time again" perceives his own experiences and his interactions with others and can alert the staff to the patient's underlying fragile capacity for mentalization. Such information can contribute to a dynamic understanding of risk with respect to the patient's interpersonal relationships. When the attachment system is stimulated or affect aroused to the point of dysregulation, non-mentalizing ways of experiencing subjective reality can predominate and violence can break through. However, an individual's capacity to mentalize varies depending upon the context and the person to whom the patient is relating and, as such, the ID consultation can only function as a non-specific indicator of compromised mentalization. What the ID consultation can achieve more effectively is getting teams to mentalize about their patients. Of course if teams can accurately and empathically keep their patients in mind, patients will feel understood. Such holding in mind can help contain affective dysregulation and minimise acting out, especially aggression. Although it is clinically appealing to postulate that completing the ID consultation, especially if the process is undertaken regularly within the team and involves consulting with the patient, may improve the patient's capacity to mentalize, to date there is no empirical evidence to support this. It may be that patient care benefits through another mechanism, namely that undertaking the ID consultation helps get elements of mentalization into team functioning. The sharing of thinking and experience about the patient necessarily involves team members considering the perspective of other members. Through this process the rigid and fixed perspectives that characterise splitting within teams may be resolved. The ID consultation fosters a non-hierarchical environment and a capacity to mentalize in a group with other team members. These aspects of mentalizing should improve team functioning, help contain risk, enhance patient-care and decrease the pull towards chaos within forensic systems.

References

Adshead, G., & Bluglass, K. (2005). Attachment representations in mothers with abnormal illness behaviour by proxy. *British Journal of Psychiatry, 187*: 328–333.

Ainsworth, M. D. S. (1967). *Infancy in Uganda: Infant Care and the Growth of Love*. Baltimore, MD: Johns Hopkins University Press.

Ainsworth, M. D. S., Blehar, M. C., Waters, E., & Wall, S. (1978). *Patterns of Attachment: A Psychological Study of the Strange Situation*. Hillsdale, NJ: Erlbaum.

Allen, J. G. (2008). Mentalizing in practice. In: G. Allen & P. Fonagy (Eds.), *Handbook of Mentalization-Based Treatment* (pp. 3–30). Chichester, UK: John Wiley.

Allen, J. G., Hauser, S. T., & Borman-Spurrell, E. (1996). Attachment theory as a framework for understanding sequelae of severe adolescent psychopathology: an 11-year follow-up study. *Journal of Consulting and Clinical Psychology, 64*: 254–263.

Allen, J. G., Lemma, A., & Fonagy, P. (2012). Trauma. In: A. W. Bateman & P. Fonagy (Eds.), *Handbook of Mentalizing in Mental Health Practice* (pp. 419–444). Washington, DC: American Psychiatric Publishing.

Babcock, J. C., Jacobson, N. S., Gottman, J. M., & Yerington, T. P. (2000). Attachment, emotional regulation and the function of marital violence: differences between secure, preoccupied and dismissing violent and nonviolent husbands. *Journal of Family Violence, 15*: 391–409.

Bakermans-Kranenburg, M. J., & van IJzendoorn, M. H. (2009). The first 10,000 Adult Attachment Interviews: distributions of adult attachment representations in clinical and non-clinical groups. *Attachment & Human Development, 11*: 223–263.

Barone, L. (2003). Developmental protective and risk factors in borderline pd: a study using the Adult Attachment Interview. *Attachment & Human Development, 5*(1): 64–77.

Benjamin, L. S. (1996). A clinician-friendly version of the interpersonal circumplex: Structural Analysis of Social Behavior (SASB). *Journal of Personality Assessment, 66*: 248–266.

Bifulco, A., Moran, P., Ball, C., & Bernazzani, O. (2002). Adult attachment style. I: Its relationship to clinical depression. *Social Psychiatry and Psychiatric Epidemiology, 37*: 50–59.

Bowlby, J. (1951). Maternal care and mental health. *Bulletin from World Health Organization*, 355–533.

Bowlby, J. (1969). Observations to be explained. In: *Attachment and Loss, Vol 1: Attachment* (pp. 46–57). London: Hogarth Press and the Institute of Psycho-Analysis.

Bowlby, J. (1973). *Attachment and Loss, Vol II: Separation: Anxiety and Anger*. New York, NY: Basic.

Bowlby, J. (1977). The making and breaking of affectional bonds. I. Aetiology and psychopathology in the light of attachment theory. An expanded version of the Fiftieth Maudsley Lecture, delivered before the Royal College of Psychiatrists, 19 November 1976, *British Journal of Psychiatry, 130*: 201–210.

Bowlby, J. (1980). *Attachment and Loss, Vol III: Loss: Sadness and Depression*. New York, NY: Basic.

Bowlby, J. (1988). *A Secure Base: Parent–Child Attachments and Healthy Human Development*. London: Routledge.

Bretherton, I. (1995). The origins of attachment theory. In: S. Goldberg, R. Muir, & J. Kerr (Eds.), *Attachment Theory, Social, Developmental and Clinical Perspectives* (pp. 45–84). Hillsdale, NJ: The Analytic Press.

Bretherton, I., & Munholland, K. A. (1999). Internal working models in attachment relationships; a construct revisited. In: J. Cassidy, & P. R. Shaver (Eds.), *Handbook of Attachment; Theory, Research and Clinical Applications* (pp. 89–111). New York, NY: Guilford Press.

Brown, G. W., & Harris, T. O. (1978). *The Social Origins of Depression: A Study of Psychiatric Disorder in Women*. London: Tavistock.

Carlson, E. A. (1998). A prospective longitudinal study of attachment disorganization/disorientation. *Child Development, 69*: 1107–1128.

Carlson, V., Cicchetti, D., Barnett, D., & Braunwald, K. (1989). Disorganized/disoriented attachment relationships in maltreated infants. *Developmental Psychology, 25*: 525–531.

Caspi, A., McClay, J., Moffitt, T. E., Mill, J., Martin, J., Craig, I. W., Taylor, A., & Poulton, R. (2002). Role of genotype in the cycle of violence in maltreated children. *Science, 297*: 851–854.

Caspi, A., Moffitt, T. E., Morgan, J., Rutter, M., Taylor, A., Arseneault, L., Tully, L., Jacobs, C., Kim-Cohen, J., & Polo-Tomas, M. (2004). Maternal expressed emotion predicts children's antisocial behavior problems: using monozygotic-twin differences to identify environmental effects on behavioral development. *Developmental Psychology, 40*: 149–161.

Caspi, A., Sugden, K., Moffitt, T. E., Taylor, A., Craig, I. W., Harrington, H., McClay, J., Mill, J., Martin, J., Braithwaite, A., & Poulton, R. (2003). Influence of life stress on depression: moderation by a polymorphism in the 5-HTT gene. *Science, 301*: 386–389.

Cassidy, J. (2008). The nature of the child's ties. In: J. Cassidy & P. R. Shaver (Eds.), *Handbook of Attachment. Theory, Research, and Clinical Applications*, 2nd edition (pp. 3–22). New York, NY: Guilford Press.

Cicchetti, D. (2004). An odyssey of discovery: lessons learned through three decades of research on child maltreatment. *American Journal of Psychology, 59*: 731–741.

Cicchetti, D., & Toth, S. (1995). A developmental psychopathology perspective on child abuse and neglect. *Journal of American Academy of Child and Adolescent Psychiatry, 34*: 541–565.

Coid, J. (1992). DSM-III diagnosis in criminal psychopaths: a way forward. *Criminal Behaviour and Mental Health, 2*: 78–94.

Cole-Detke, H., & Kobak, R. (1996). Attachment processes in eating disorder and depression, *Journal of Consulting and Clinical Psychology, 64*: 282–290.

Crittenden, P. M. (2000). A dynamic-maturational approach to continuity and change in pattern of attachment. In: P. M. Crittenden & A. H. Claussen (Eds.), *The Organisation of Attachment Relationships: Maturation, Culture, and Context* (pp. 343–357). New York, NY: Cambridge University Press.

Crittenden, P. M., Partridge, M. F., & Claussen, A. H. (1991). Family patterns of relationship in normative and dysfunctional families. *Development and Psychopathology, 3*: 491–512.

Davies, P. T., Cummings, E. M., & Winter, M. A. (2004). Pathways between profiles of family functioning, child security in the interparental subsystem, and child psychological problems. *Development and Psychopathology, 16*: 525–550.

DeKlyen, M., & Greenberg, M. T. (2008). Attachment and psychopathology in childhood. In: J. Cassidy & P. R. Shaver (Eds.), *Handbook of Attachment. Theory, Research, and Clinical Applications*, 2nd edition (pp. 637–665). New York, NY: Guilford Press.

De Rosnay, M., & Harris, P. L. (2002). Individual differences in children's understanding of emotion: The roles of attachment and language. *Attachment and Human Development, 4*: 39–54.

Dozier, M., Cue, K. L., & Barnett, L. (1994). Clinicians as caregivers: role of attachment organization in treatment. *Journal of Consulting and Clinical Psychology, 62:* 793–800.

Fonagy, P. (2003a). The interpersonal interpretive mechanism—the confluence of genetics and attachment theory in development. In: V. Green (Ed.), *Emotional Development in Psychoanalysis, Attachment and Neuroscience: Creating Connections* (pp. 107–126). London: Karnac.

Fonagy, P. (2003b). Towards a developmental understanding of violence. *British Journal of Psychiatry, 183*: 190–192.

Fonagy, P., Bateman, A. W., Luyten, P. (2012). Introduction and overview. In: A. W. Bateman & P. Fonagy (Eds.), *Handbook of Mentalizing in Mental Health Practice* (pp. 3–42). Washington, DC: American Psychiatric Publishing, Inc.

Fonagy, P., Leigh, T., Steele, M., Steele, H., Kennedy, R., Mattoon, G., Target, M., & Gerber, A. (1996). The relation of attachment status, psychiatric classification, and response to psychotherapy. *Journal of Consulting and Clinical Psychology, 64*(1): 22–31.

Fonagy, P., Luyten, P., & Strathearn, I. (2011). Borderline personality disorder, mentalization, and the neurobiology of attachment. *Infant Mental Health Journal, 32:* 47–69.

Fonagy, P., Steele, M., Steele, H., Moran, G. S., & Higgitt, A. C. (1991). The capacity for understanding mental states: The reflective self in parent and child and its significance for security of attachment. *Infant Mental Health Journal, 12*: 201–218.

Fonagy, P., Target, M., Steele, M., Steele, H., Leigh, T., Levinson, A., & Kennedy, R. (1997). Morality, disruptive behaviour, borderline Pd, crime and their relationships to security of attachment. In: L. Atkinson & K. J. Zucker, (Eds.), *Attachment and Psychopathology* (pp. 223–274). New York, NY: Guilford Press.

Freud, S. (1957). Five lectures on psychoanalysis. In: J. Stachey (Ed. & Trans.), *The Standard Edition of the Complete Psychological Works of Sigmund Freud* (Vol. 23) (pp. 139–207). London: Hogarth Press.

Frodi, A., Dernevik, M., Sepa, A., Philipson, J., & Bragesjo, M. (2001). Current attachment representations of incarcerated offenders varying in degree of psychopathy. *Attachment Human Development, 3*: 269–283.

George, C., Kaplan, N., & Main, M. (1996). *The Adult Attachment Interview (3rd edition)*. Berkeley, CA: Department of Psychology, University of California at Berkeley. Unpublished Work.

Harlow, H. F. (1958). The nature of love. *American Psychologist, 13*: 673–685.

Harris, T., Brown, G. W., & Bifulco, A. (1986). Loss of parent in childhood and adult psychiatric disorder: the role of lack of adequate parental care. *Psychological Medicine, 16*: 641–659.

Hesse, E. (1996). Discourse, memory, and the adult attachment interview: A note with emphasis on the emerging cannot classify category. *Infant Mental Health, 17*: 4–11.

Holtzworth-Munroe, A., Stuart, G. L., & Hutchinson, G. (1997). Violent versus nonviolent husbands: differences in attachment patterns, dependency and jealousy. *Journal of Family Psychology, 11*: 314–331.

Insel, T. R., & Winslow, J. T. (2004). The neurobiology of social attachment. In: D. S. Charney & E. J. Nestler (Eds.), *Neurobiology of Mental Illness*, 2nd edition (pp. 1101–1111). Oxford: Oxford University Press.

Kandel, E. R. (1998). A new intellectual framework for psychiatry. *American Journal of Psychiatry, 155*: 457–469.

Kendler, K. S. (2005). "A gene for …": the nature of gene action in psychiatric disorders. *American Journal of Psychiatry, 162*: 1243–1252.

Kobak, R., Cassidy, J., Lyons-Ruth, K., & Ziv, Y. (2006). Attachment, stress, and psychopathology: A developmental pathways model. In: D. Cicchetti & D. J. Cohen (Eds.), *Developmental Psychopathology: Volume One: Theory and Method*, Second edition (pp. 333–367). New Jersey, NJ: John Wiley & Sons.

Koren-Karie, N., Oppenheim, D., Dolev, S., Sher, E., & Etzion-Carasso, A. (2002). Mothers' insightfulness regarding their infants' internal experience: relations with maternal sensitivity and infant attachment. *Developmental Psychopathology, 38*: 534–542.

Levinson, A., & Fonagy, P. (2004). Offending and attachment: the relationship between interpersonal awareness and offending in a prison population with psychiatric disorder. *Canadian Journal of Psychoanalysis, 12*: 225–251.

Lorenz, K. E. (1935). Der Kumpan in der Umvelt des Vogels. *Journal of Ornithology, 83*: 137–213, 289–413.

Luyten, P., Fonagy, P., Lowyck, B., Vermote, R. (2012). Assessment of mentalization. In: A. W. Bateman & P. Fonagy (Eds.), *Handbook of Mentalizing in Mental Health Practice* (pp. 43–65). Washington, DC: American Psychiatric Publishing.

Lyons-Ruth, K., Alpern, L., & Repacholi, B. (1993). Disorganized infant attachment classification and maternal psychosocial problems as predictors of hostile-aggressive behavior in the preschool classroom. *Child Development, 64*: 572–585.

Main, M., & Hesse, E. (1990). Parents' unresolved traumatic experiences are related to infant disorganized attachment status: Is frightened and/or frightening parental behavior the linking mechanism. In: M. T. Greenberg, D. Cicchetti, & E. M. Cummings (Eds.), *Attachment in the Preschool Years. Theory, Research, and Intervention* (pp. 161–182). Chicago, IL: University of Chicago Press.

Main, M. & Hesse, E. (1992). Frightening, frightened, dissociated, or disorganized behavior on the part of the parent: A coding system for parent–infant interactions. Berkeley, CA: University of California at Berkeley. Unpublished manuscript.

Main, M. & Solomon, J. (1989). Procedures for identifying infants as disorganized disoriented during the ainsworth strange situation. In: M. T. Greenberg, D. Cicchetti, & E. M. Cummings (Eds.), *Attachment in the Preschool Years. Theory, Research, and Intervention* (pp. 121–159). Chicago, IL: University of Chicago Press.

Main, M., Goldwyn, R., & Hesse, E. (2003). Adult attachment scoring and classification system. Berkeley, CA: Department of Psychology, University of California at Berkeley. Unpublished work.

Manassis, K., Bradley, S., Goldberg, S., Hood, J., & Swinson, R. P. (1994). Attachment in mothers with anxiety disorders and their children. *Journal of the American Academy of Child and Adolescent Psychiatry, 33*: 1106–1113.

McGauley, G., Yakeley, J., Williams, A., & Bateman, A. (2011). Attachment, mentalization and antisocial personality disorder; the possible contribution of mentalization-based treatment. *European Journal of Psychotherapy and Counselling, 13*: 1–23.

McGuffin, P., Riley, B., & Plomin, R. (2001). Genomics and behavior. Toward behavioral genomics. *Science, 291*: 1232–1249.

Munson, J. A., McMahon, R. J., & Spieker, S. J. (2001). Structure and variability in the developmental trajectory of children's externalizing problems:

impact of infant attachment, maternal depressive symptomatology, and child sex. *Developmental Psychopathology, 13*: 277–296.

Muris, P., & Meesters, C. (2002). Attachment, behavioral inhibition, and anxiety disorders symptoms in normal adolescents. *Journal of Psychopathology and Behavioral Assessment, 24*: 97–106.

Muris, P., Mayer, B., & Meesters, C. (2000). Self-reported attachment style, anxiety, and depression in children. *Social Behavior and Personality, 28*: 157–162.

O'Connor, T. (2006). The persisting effects of early experiences on psychological development. In: D. Cicchetti & D. J. Cohen (Eds.), *Developmental Psychopathology, Vol II*, 2nd edition (pp. 202–234). Chichester, UK: John Wiley & Sons.

O'Connor, T. G., Marvin, R. S., Rutter, M., Olrick, J. T., & Britner, P. A. (2003). Child-parent attachment following early institutional deprivation. *Developmental Psychopathology, 15*(1): 19–38.

Patrick, M., Hobson, R. P., Castle, D., Howard, R., & Maughan, B. (1994). Personality disorder and the mental representation of early social experience. *Development and Psychopathology, 6*: 375–388.

Pert, L., Ferriter, M., & Saul, C. (2004). Parental loss before the age of 16 years: a comparative study of patients with personality disorder and patients with schizophrenia in a high secure hospital's population. *Psychology and Psychotherapy: Theory, Research and Practice, 77*: 403–407.

Plomin, R., & Bergeman, C. S. (1991). The nature of nurture: genetic influence on "environmental" measures. *Behavioral and Brain Sciences, 14*: 373–427.

Rosenstein, D. S. & Horowitz, H. A. (1996). Adolescent attachment and psychopathology, *Journal of Consulting and Clinical Psychology, 64:* 244–253.

Rutter, M. (1971). Parent–child separation: psychological effects on the children. *Journal of Child Psychology and sychiatry, 12*: 233–260.

Rutter, M. (2004). The psychological effects of early institutional rearing. In: P. Marshall & N. Fox (Eds.), *The Development of Social Engagement: Neurobiological Perspectives* (pp. 355–392). Oxford: Oxford University Press.

Rutter, M. (2005a). How the environment affects mental health. *British Journal of Psychiatry, 186*: 4–6.

Rutter, M. (2005b). Environmentally mediated risks for psychopathology: research strategies and findings. *Journal of the American Academy of Child and Adolescent Psychiatry, 44*(1): 3–18.

Rutter, M., Kreppner, J., & O'Connor, T. G. (2001). The english and romanian adoptees study team, specificity and hererogeneity in children's responses to profound privation. *British Journal of Psychiatry, 179*: 97–103.

Rutter, M., Silberg, J., O'Connor, T., & Simonoff, E. (1999). Genetics and child psychiatry: I advances in quantitative and molecular genetics. *Journal of Child Psychology and Psychiatry, 40*(1): 3–18.

Sroufe, L. A. (2005). Attachment and development: a prospective, longitudinal study from birth to adulthood. *Attachment and Human Development, 7*: 349–367.

Sroufe, L. A., Carlson, E. A., Levy, A. K., & Egeland, B. (1999). Implications of attachment theory for developmental psychopathology. *Developmental Psychopathology, 11*(1): 1–13.

Steele, M. (2003). Attachment, actual experience and mental representation. In: V. Green (Ed.), *Emotional Development in Psychoanalysis, Attachment Theory and Neuroscience. Creating Connections* (pp. 86–106). New York, NY: Brunner Routledge.

Tyrrell, C. L., Dozier, M., Teague, G. B., & Fallot, R. D. (1999). Effective treatment relationships for persons with serious psychiatric disorders: the importance of attachment states of mind. *Journal of Consulting and Clinical Psychology, 67*: 725–733.

Van Emmichoven, I. A. Z., van IJzendoorn, M. H., de Ruiter, C., & Brosschot, J. F. (2003). Selective processing of threatening information: effects of attachment representation and anxiety disorder on attention and memory. *Development and Psychopathology, 15*(1): 219–237.

van IJzendoorn, M. H., & Bakermans-Kranenburg, M. J. (1996). Attachment representations in mothers, fathers, adolescents, and clinical groups: a meta-analytic search for normative data. *Journal of Consulting and Clinical Psychology, 64*(1): 8–21.

van IJzendoorn, M. H., & Bakermans-Kranenburg, M. J. (1997). Intergenerational transmission of attachment: A move to the contextual level. In: L. Atkinson & K. J. Zucker (Eds.), *Attachment and Psychopathology* (pp. 135–170). New York, NY: Guilford Press.

van IJzendoorn, M. H., Feldbrugge, J. T., Derks, F. C., de Ruiter, C., Verhagen, M. F., Philipse, M. W., van der Staak, C. P., & Riksen-Walraven, J. M. (1997). Attachment representations of personality-disordered criminal offenders. *American Journal of Orthopsychiatry, 67*: 449–459.

Ward, A., Ramsay, R., Turnbull, S., Steele, M., Steele, H., & Treasure, J. (2001). Attachment in anorexia nervosa: a transgenerational perspective. *British Journal of Medical Psychology, 74*: 497–505.

Winnicott, D. W. (1963). Morals and education. In: *The Maturational Processes and the Facilitating Environment* (pp. 93–105). London: Hogarth Press.

Yakeley, J. (2014). Mentalization-based group treatment for antisocial personality disorder. In: *Forensic Group Psychotherapy. The Portman Papers* (pp. 151–182). London: Karnac.

CHAPTER THREE

Perverse states of mind and perverse enactment: the ID consultation in a case of paraphilia

Maggie McAlister

The Interpersonal Dynamics (ID) consultation is particularly useful for facilitating a focused and structured clinical discussion where the purpose is to elucidate dysfunctional patterns of relationship that can impede progress and threaten to derail treatment plans and therapeutic engagement. The focus of the consultation is to bring to light interactions that cause great difficulty for the treatment team but are often difficult to pinpoint or to bring together in a coherent whole, given that a persistent feature of our client group is a tendency to fragment both internally and in their relationships. An ID consultation can throw into relief pervasive patterns of relationship within the client's inner world and show how these interactions may have been present within the index offence and persist via transference to the current treatment setting. This can then be very helpful for formulating scenarios for the HCR-20 risk assessment protocol (Webster, Douglas, Eaves, & Hart, 1997) alongside overall treatment planning.

A central feature of the client group in a medium secure setting is that the index offence has involved a severe form of acting out; there has been a wish to evacuate an intolerable state of mind through the offending behaviour. This is perhaps more immediately apparent in the case of violent offences. What may be more difficult to spot are those offences of a perverse nature where deception, denial, and splitting are particularly involved. Through the lens of Glasser's (1986) psychoanalytic theory of the core complex, in this chapter I intend to explore aspects of perversion where the care itself is perverted.

Understanding the dynamics

A core feature of forensic patients is how thinking can be replaced with action. This is most clearly illustrated in the form of the offending behaviour. The emphasis is on action as opposed to thought, due to a deficit in the capacity to think or reflect especially in moments of strong emotional arousal or anxiety. The means by which offenders discharge anxiety is to "act out". This is central to how, as psychotherapists, we understand their offending as an unconscious enactment of an earlier conflict which arouses intense anxiety and needs to be evacuated through physical action.

What we understand to be acted out is an unbearable state of mind in order to maintain power or control. One of the internal splits this can create is that between the victim and the perpetrator states of mind. We often see this in our client group, where patients become identified with either one pole of experience or the other: either seeing themselves as hardened aggressors (as a defence against their vulnerability) or as blameless victims of others or the Criminal Justice System (as a defence against the damage they inflict on others). The perpetrator maintains psychic equilibrium and evacuates an intolerable state of mind into the other. It is this state of mind that we are often mindful of capturing in the ID consultation where defences such as projective identification come into play. What we have repeatedly found in consulting to teams using the ID approach is that there is often an enactment between the patient and the treatment team of the dynamics around the index offence, which in turn is itself often a re-enactment of an earlier trauma in the patient's life. As well as the past returning into the present, one can also predict scenarios of risk for the future based on historical and clinical evidence.

The perverse state of mind

In the context of this paper, what is meant by a perverse state of mind is a state of disavowal, the paradox of both knowing something and not knowing it. Steiner (1985) has used the term "turning a blind eye" for a defence that is characteristic of a distortion and misrepresentation of reality. This particular kind of defence arises from what Glasser (1986) has called the "core complex", a particular constellation of anxieties and defences which come into being in early infancy and become a fixation point for the individual. The core complex describes a fixed mode of relating which seeks to bind or control contact with the other in order to avoid total annihilation (engulfment) on the one hand or total isolation (abandonment) on the other. Glasser traces this mode of relating to the individual's earliest relationship with his mother where the relationship is characterised by excessive intrusiveness, alternating with neglect, withdrawal, and abandonment. It is a relationship from which there is no escape—the infant is utterly dependent on the caregiver—and furthermore there is often an absent father, no "third other" who could provide triangulation into an alternative space/relationship. In order to manage these irreconcilable conflicts, the individual develops a mode of relating that avoids true intimacy, based on sadomasochistic control, distortions of reality, simulation (as opposed to true identification) and deception, where the true self is kept hidden and inviolate. Glasser saw the core complex as being at the heart of all perversions and viewed all offending as a perversion of relatedness and intimacy.

Sadomasochistic violence differs from other types of violence (self-preservative, psychotic, and rage type violence) in important ways. In sadomasochistic violence, the ongoing relationship to the object is paramount—the object must be seen to suffer. Furthermore the violence is *considered*, and there is an absence of anxiety (pleasure is present). In contrast, self-preservative violence is triggered by danger and tends to be directed at eliminating the threat. It is accompanied by eruptive affect: anxiety followed by relief. Essentially, sadomasochistic relating aims to "bind" the object, preserve its continuing existence and inflict ongoing or repeated suffering.

Features of the core complex:

- Rigid, obsessive control of the other
- Continuing involvement but avoidance of true intimacy
- Sadomasochism: contact with the other but in specifically controlled situations dominated by violence, cruelty, and pain.

Characteristics of perversion:

- Anxiety (perversion binds and contains profound anxiety)
- Deception
- Denial of difference (e.g., differences between generations)

- Splitting and part object relating (not seeing others as whole persons with separate minds and bodies)
- Sadism (sexualisation of aggression)
- Attempt at a reversal of experience, where the perpetrator evacuates their own experience into others by creating fear, vulnerability, and loss in the victim.

Examples of perversions:

- Trans-generational relationships involving sexual abuse of the young
- Fetishism—the idealisation of substance over human involvement
- Exhibitionism/voyeurism
- Reversal of paranoid fears using protective identification
- Criminal activities attacking life, sexuality or property as in violence, rape, and theft.

For any index offence one could expect some of the above characteristics to be present in the interpersonal dynamics between the service user and staff team. However, for those involving a sexual perversion, elements of distortion, misrepresentation of reality, sadistic control, denial, and deception may become significant issues in the dynamics involved. I shall now focus on clinical material to explore these issues further.

The following case study is of an ID consultation I conducted abroad in a forensic service following my attendance at an international conference. The case has been heavily disguised and drawn from a composite of consultations of a similar nature in order to protect confidentiality without losing any of the salient features of the case.

Mr G

Mr G, a man in his early thirties, was on a rehab ward in medium security following his conviction of charges of sexual harassment of a nine-year-old girl, the daughter of his partner at the time of the offence. Mr G received a hospital order at sentencing and rapidly settled down to life on the unit. On the one hand he was very settled and calm in his interactions, but on the other he put tremendous pressure on professionals for his discharge, stating that he did not need to be detained as he had full insight into his offence and had made a full recovery from a "touch of schizophrenia". He appeared fairly intact with no reports of any psychotic experiences, and he had been on a drug free trial for many months. However, although calm and reasonable, he created heightened tension in staff, and to sit with him was often unbearable due to the intense anxiety one felt in his presence. He was vehemently emphatic that he needed to be discharged as quickly as possible.

A difficult pattern of interaction developed where Mr G disengaged from any therapeutic engagement, and staff began to struggle with his constant demands. These mainly took the form of demands for a tribunal and an absolute discharge. However, there were other continual demands: nothing on the ward in his daily care was ever good enough, and staff constantly felt undermined and criticised in their attempts to attend to him. Added to this, professional reports were often found wanting, to the extent that Mr G would examine the meaning and connotation of every word, dismissing professional opinion and threatening litigation. This meant ward staff were often pulled in to his constant demands in a way that was disabling and time consuming. One felt taken hostage by his needs and that one's hand was being forced. Amongst all of this, there was also a way in which Mr G rallied other patients into his complaints after which he would take a back seat and watch things escalate on the ward. Staff often felt terrified of facing a riot in which Mr G always felt like a peripheral figure. He also seemed to be at the centre of many dealings on the ward and to take a special position with his peers. It would come to light that he would acquire new possessions by bartering with fellow service users in an exploitative and ruthless manner (e.g., acquiring an MP3 player by offering to buy a more vulnerable fellow service user a Chinese takeaway). Illicit substances soon started to become a problem on the ward, and staff began to suspect that Mr G was drug dealing.

In our discussion, it also came to light that staff could see situations where they had compromised their boundaries or their usual way of doing things. For example, one staff member spoke about ways in which Mr G could get her to talk about herself in a more personal way than she would normally, especially when escorting him on leave in the grounds. This boundary slippage seemed to arise partly in response to his constant demands and his sense of special entitlement, but also partly something else: a feeling of guilt and sympathy, as if one was being too punitive, rejecting, and restricting by asserting a boundary in the first place. In this sense he became increasingly difficult to say no to, despite staff feeling aware of how uncomfortable this made them.

On the whole, the multidisciplinary team felt worn down. However, in our discussion what emerged was another strand to the interactions. What if he were right? What if he were the victim of a miscarriage of justice? What if he was just attempting to help the girl, and it all became misconstrued and misinterpreted? The man may be innocent of all charges. He doesn't have an illness—maybe we should let him go …

Historical factors

Some significant historical factors in Mr G's background are worth highlighting regarding both his later index offence and his pervasive patterns of relating on the ward. During his mother's pregnancy with him, his father disappeared leaving Mr G fatherless and his mother alone during his upbringing, a remote farm in the middle of rural countryside. Mr G had an older brother and sister, and it is believed that they were involved in raising the patient from a young age. During his early adolescence, his mother left him in the care of his brother as she moved elsewhere.

In his late teens, he left the farm and found temporary accommodation in a nearby city. He then worked in several manual jobs during which time he developed a serious drug habit and started using crack cocaine and heroin. He acquired a criminal record—including convictions for drug offences and driving offences. Around this time, Mr G took a trip abroad. Mr G's account is that when he was returning, he bumped into some friends who offered to give him a lift in their van. He was in the van while the others had gone to get some food, and the police arrived, searched the van and found illegal immigrants stowed away in the back. Mr G was arrested and charged for this and spent several years in a foreign prison. Following his return he managed to secure a job as a truck driver in spite of developing dependency on heroin. He lost his job after he had some peripheral involvement in a hostage taking incident during which a security guard was shot dead. He claims to have been forced at gunpoint by an acquaintance and his associates to rent a car that was subsequently used in the kidnapping.

The index offence

Mr G had started a relationship with a woman whom he met through work. She was heavily pregnant at the time and had other children. Mr G stated that it was "love at first sight". He moved in with her and even helped deliver her baby. He later spoke about this being a very strong part of the attraction for him, the fact that she had children who needed to be provided for and looked after, especially the baby boy. He stated that there were times when he put up with tension in the relationship in order to continue his contact with the children. However, in time he started expressing unusual thoughts about the nine-year-old daughter. His partner's account to the police was that he became obsessed with her and started to tell her that he was in love with her. At one point, he climbed through her first floor window in order to tell her that he loved her. His partner phoned the police, and he was told not to return to the property.

Nevertheless, after several days he returned to the flat. The police eventually came, and a psychiatric assessment was arranged. He was taken to a nearby hospital but discharged quite quickly and returned for the second time to the property a day or so later. He was turned away by his partner's brother, but he yet again returned the next day proclaiming his love for the girl, having written her a love letter.

A week later, he had gone to her school and approached her, grabbing her arm and telling her that he loved her. The police were called, and he was arrested and taken to the police station.

He was remanded to custody, and when assessed by his catchment area forensic psychiatrist Mr G presented as depressed and withdrawn. He also displayed disturbed behaviour in that he would try and run away from his cell and had to be restrained regularly. He was still preoccupied with his victim, believing that there were messages from the TV saying that he should go ahead and marry her.

Following his admission to the medium secure unit, Mr G's psychotic beliefs about his love affair with the girl quickly subsided, and he recognised that he was ill at the time, saying that it all felt "like a dream".

The four interpersonal perspectives

In meeting with the team, the brief formulation of the four perspectives went as follows:

Perspective A

Mr G repeatedly experiences others as **depending** on him (his ex-partner, fellow service users). He has a tendency to experience persons in authority as **accusing** him and **controlling** him. He also feels that staff are **ignoring** his needs such as his repeated requests to meet his family in hospital grounds and his repeated complaints that there is nothing for him to do on the ward.

Perspective B

Mr G experiences himself as greatly **attending to and caring** as evidenced in his previous relationship and also in his account of his childhood relationship with his mother where he felt he had to protect and look after her. He also rationalised his behaviour with regard to the index offence, denied his sexual attraction for an underage girl and justified his behaviour as "saving her life". On the ward he sees himself as protective and helpful to other patients, often resulting in conflict with staff because he is seen as interfering in the care of others and encouraging dissent and complaints. He **treats himself as special**, expressing a somewhat idealised view of himself by stating that there should be different rules for him as there is nothing wrong with him.

If his idealised view of himself is challenged he is **self-justifying**, angrily attacking his care and making threats, with occasional acts of violence such as throwing a hot drink at a nurse whom he believed had slighted him in some way. Alternatively, if he complies with demands, he can experience himself as **appeasing and complying** with authority.

Perspective C

In response others experience Mr G as **domineering and imposing** (controlling staff suspiciously, demanding that his needs are immediately met), **intimidating and attacking** them if they do not meet his needs, and also **exploiting and manipulating** them (e.g., intrusive demands upon his victim, drug dealing on the ward, exploitation of his peers, getting staff to break boundaries). Staff perceive him as **behaving as though he knows best**, insisting on his view of events and attempting to dictate his care.

Perspective D

As a consequence staff and others feel they are constantly **appeasing and complying** (careful how they write reports or respond to his unreasonable request for a high tech games console) or otherwise **defying and**

opposing him when they don't give in to his demands. In response to his demands and persistent requests, staff feel they are **fleeing** from him (like the young victim literally had to do) and at times as **rejecting him** due to a wish to avoid him. Alternatively, they can also get caught up in an idealised view, where he is **accepted and admired**. This is expressed in the feelings of guilt and sympathy—a feeling that one is perhaps being too rigid and treating him in an excessively unfair manner.

The basic formulation and the core complex

The pattern of feelings and interactions discerned in this ID basic formulation is indicative of the dynamics we could expect from the core complex. There are repeated patterns of idealisation and dependency (portending engulfment) alternating with rejection and exclusion (abandonment). However, even the experience of accepting and admiring him (Perspective D) has a quality of abandonment within it, as it can lead staff to turn a blind eye or be willing to overlook boundary breaches and, consequently, to ignore Mr G's real needs. Essentially, the emotional quality of the relationship is one of sadistic control, manipulation, and deception, and the core complex oscillation is between merger on the one hand (appeasing/complying/accepting/admiring) or abandonment on the other (avoidance/rejection/withdrawal). Furthermore there is a pervading sense of impasse: one is either controlling him or being controlled. The experience staff have of wishing to ignore him/flee from him/reject him feeds into the perception Mr G has of others accusing/controlling and ignoring him, whereas the more "merged" experiences of appeasing/complying/admiring feed into the perception Mr G has of others depending on him (Perspective A). Thus a vicious cycle is created, and the circle begins again.

Past, present, future … The extended formulation

Mr G's early exposure to trauma was in the form of his father's disappearance prior to his birth. Growing up without his father, he stated how he felt he had to become his mother's partner/saviour and had a role of feeling he had to take care of her. The subsequent trauma he experienced was his later abandonment by his mother where he was left in the care of his older siblings in early adolescence. This process links with his assumed role within the family in relation to the index offence in which he distorted reason in a psychotic state of mind and made a claim for the right to marry a nine-year-old girl—the more needy parts of himself (which were intolerable to him) projectively identified into the victim. Consequently, his attempts to save/protect her by offering to marry her represented an unconscious attempt to save/protect himself.

These patterns of being a saviour (the mother, the partner, the young girl, his fellow service users) could all be examples of ways in which he deals with his own loss and vulnerability by unconsciously attributing it to others. He also fulfils the role of the "great helper" on the ward, recreating his role in the family which he exploited and abused in a perverse state of mind which also perhaps is enacted through his role as a human trafficker. Professionals experience him as exerting sadistic control of others in his interactions; one feels either massively intruded into or kept at arm's length: an identification with his image of his mother as aggressor. When the ward staff authority is asserted, he adjusts and submits in a somewhat passive way, simulating a sense of himself as a "victim". This victim state of mind is seen time and again in his "innocent" involvement in criminal activities and in his bystander status on the ward, where he is often on the periphery of disturbances and volatile events.

In terms of the ID cycle, his early pattern of being abandoned by his parents seems to be repeated in the way that he generates feelings in others of either controlling him suspiciously or wanting to flee from him. This he achieves by telling everyone that nothing is good enough for him and making others feel that they are neglecting his needs. This can result in enactments where others, out of a sense of guilt, find themselves making special allowances and being pressured to behave in unusual or out of the ordinary ways. Others also find themselves turning a blind eye to how disturbed Mr G is by questioning his diagnosis and treatment needs. In all of these enactments there are elements of deception and disavowal.

Implications for treatment and outcomes

A central challenge for staff managing the care of Mr G can be described in terms of the "autonomy/control" axis of the ID circumplex (see Chapter One). In discussion, they found that his view was that you are either with me or against me; the temptation was either to give in or to control—or to avoid contact with Mr G in an attempt to evade the dilemma. Staff also identified that he saw any boundary or restriction as control, and yet they themselves were the ones feeling truly submissive, harassed, and held hostage to his demands. Staff members felt controlled in both their *thinking* (a powerful restriction in feely expressing professional opinions in report writing and meetings, for example) and in their *actions* (carrying out ordinary care planning and clinical interventions). By identifying some of these perverse enactments and distortions to ordinary care and treatment, my hope was that the ID consultation would pave the way for greater professional freedom and decision-making.

We identified three main points from the ID consultation which were relevant to the care plan for Mr G. In terms of the core complex, these areas cover the dimensions of being merged with one's object (losing one's identity and sense of self through being overwhelmed and engulfed by the other); cutting off contact (withdrawal and abandonment); and finally the sadomasochistic retreat/defence. The three main points were as follows:

1. *Merger*
    - An awareness of a tendency to take an idealised view.

      Staff discussed ways in which it could be difficult at times to hold on to an independent judgement due to Mr G's tendency to play the "innocent victim". Staff also discussed the danger of taking a minimised view of his disturbance, and some further thought was given to the care plan regarding staff members who could be isolated by Mr G (escorts, for example) who might be put under pressure regarding boundary breaking/bending, which previously had been the case. Staff also discussed the importance of the need for "ordinary" treatment, that is, a need to beware of "special case" decisions. This point addressed the tendency to view Mr G as a special case, for whom exceptions should be made. In essence, this reflects being completely taken over—engulfed—in a countertransference repetition of one attribute of the core complex. Although service users' needs are unique and individual, there was some recognition of certain decisions that had been taken which were not based on usual clinical practice. These were reviewed in the care plan.
2. *Withdrawal*
    - An awareness of the wish to flee from him.

      The team identified many ways in which staff members attempted to avoid Mr G physically, but also emotionally—leading at times to turning a blind eye to certain difficulties (boundary breaking for example) as a way to avoid further contact. Staff members also spoke about ways in which they actively avoided him as a way to manage the extreme feelings of anxiety they felt in his presence. This adoption of isolation as a defence particularly against murderous impulses is another fundamental aspect of the core complex, again enacted in the countertransference.

3. *Sadomasochistic defence*
    - An awareness of sadomasochistic control and coercive relating which operates as a defence against the above two oscillations, and keeps the object "bound" in a perverse enactment.

      The sadomasochistic defence in this case involves the aspects of the interpersonal dynamic based on relating through the use of control and coercion. The defence was not only in Mr G's mode of relating to the staff, but also vice versa, in the staff's relating to Mr G. We revisited aspects of the care plan which were felt to reflect this dimension of control and review alternative interventions. Further thought was given to the care plan regarding the management of Mr G's constant demands and unreasonable requests, so that these could be considered fully in a thoughtful and engaged manner, involving a team approach and MDT decision-making, with full awareness of the tendency to enact the third component of the core complex, sadomasochistic domination.

A great difficulty for staff members was freeing themselves from what felt like a punitive stance and not enacting an experience of abandonment by neglecting Mr G's real needs. By having a stronger sense of boundaries reinforced and held within the team, staff members felt freer in their interactions with Mr G. This led to some noticeable changes in his treatment as staff members became aware of the formulation and were able to recognise a difficult interpersonal dynamic based on power and control. As staff felt more able to implement boundaries and treatment decisions in a non-punitive manner, Mr G began to settle down and become less hostile and resistant to treatment decisions regarding medication, leave, etc. Mr G became more able to tolerate relationships in which he was neither destroying nor being destroyed and was accordingly more able to relinquish his default position of sadistic control.

References

Glasser, M. (1986). Identification and its vicissitudes as observed in the perversions. *International Journal of Psychoanalysis, 67*: 9–16.

Steiner, J. (1985). Turning a blind eye: The cover up for Oedipus. *International Review of Psychoanalysis, 12*: 161–172.

Webster, C. D., Douglas, K. S., Eaves, D., & Hart, S. D. (1997). *The HCR-20: Assessing the Risk for Violence. Version* 2. Lutz, FL: Psychological Assessment Resources Inc.

CHAPTER FOUR

An individualised approach to using the ID consultation: elucidation of psychosis

Ronald Doctor

In this chapter I illustrate how the Interpersonal Dynamics (ID) consultation method may be adapted by individual clinicians to think about clinical material. This individual application may be used when a staff team consultation is difficult to arrange or in between regular multidisciplinary group consultations, but it primarily functions as a structured framework which enables the mental health professional to reflect on his patients: an exemplification of the mentalizing process elaborated in Chapter Two. When combined with clinical risk assessment and management based on a psychodynamic modality, Doctor (2003) such an approach forms a sensitive radar which may not only help detect early warning signs or problems but can also provide insight into changes in a patient's functioning. The formulation of patient–staff relationship patterns can then be shared and discussed with colleagues and may facilitate interventions which head off potentially challenging or violent behaviour.

The psychoanalytic perspective (see below) has contributed to an elucidation of psychosis, and Bion's (1957) concepts of non-psychotic and psychotic parts of the personality are particularly relevant. The non-psychotic part of the personality is able to perceive reality, even though painful experiences may elicit defences which repress or transform the emotional meanings of those experiences in order to make them more bearable for the individual concerned. The key attribute is that meaning, although distorted more or less, is preserved. The psychotic part of the personality, on the other hand, is dedicated solely to the total obliteration of perceptions, emotional experiences, and thoughts which threaten to overwhelm the individual. Evacuation of all potential emotional meaning is the absolute priority for the subject who feels imminently at risk of total annihilation. The psychotic part of the personality can be so in the ascendancy that little communication is possible with the non-psychotic part of the patient, which holds an awareness of the individual's real struggles and problems even in the disguised form typical of dreams.

Faced with this radical bifurcation of the personality of their patient, staff inevitably respond by taking sides and becoming either the ideal or the murderously persecuting object according to whether they accept and relate to the psychotic or the non-psychotic part, respectively. The dilemma for staff is that if they ally themselves with the non-psychotic awareness of the patient's problems, they come to represent the annihilating contact with emotional and external reality and, thus, put themselves at risk of being attacked by the patient in the same way that he attacks the part of himself which recognises reality. Members of the professional team who attempt to sustain this fraught position can come into conflict with others who adopt the position of total disavowal advocated by the psychotic part of the personality and so fit in with the patient's view that nothing is wrong with him: all problems are outside the self. Consequently, the severe splitting, really fragmentation, within the patient's personality is reiterated within the multidisciplinary team (Darnley, Doctor, Gordon, & Kirtchuk, 2011). In this context, the individual use of the ID approach is above all a method to restore lost meaning, even when this is beyond the patient's grasp, and to recover the equilibrium necessary to establish a more integrated picture of the patient and thus become more available to the patient as a containing object.

Psychoanalytic contributions to understanding psychosis

Psychosis can be conceptualised as a lifelong battle between psychotic and non-psychotic parts of the personality. Lucas' (2009) important contribution to this was to coin the phrase "tuning into the psychotic wavelength" which succinctly encapsulated the task of trying to differentiate which part of the personality one was dealing with. Furthermore, he highlighted how difficult this task could be and how it was quite possible for the psychotic part of the personality to try to impersonate the non-psychotic part so that one could be duped into feeling that one was dealing with a rational and sane part of the personality instead (Lucas, 2009).

In my work as a forensic psychotherapist I have found these conceptualisations an invaluable aid in helping me try to decipher the severe psychotic illnesses I encounter in my daily clinical practice. The forensic task is especially difficult as our patients not only suffer from severe psychotic illnesses but, in addition, often have severe personality disorders. Furthermore, and quite crucially, they have committed terrible crimes, the sort that are counter-transferentially "hard to stomach" such is the immediate evacuative somatic response to such horrors. They are so difficult to comprehend that they cannot be borne in mind. It is not surprising that our patients have little interest in knowing anything about their crimes or the illnesses and personal histories that provide the dynamic contextual backdrop to the situation that they find themselves in.

Freud (1911a) considered psychosis a two stage process in which there was a "psychic catastrophe", characterised by a "denial or disavowal" (Freud, 1911a, p. 70) of unacceptable reality, followed by the creation of a substitute reality in the form of delusions and hallucinations to "make good the damage done" (Freud, 1924, p. 151). Freud emphasised that many of the symptoms of psychosis arose from attempts on the part of the patient to restore his damaged ego and to reconstitute a world which had been destroyed: "The delusional formation which we take to be the pathological product, is in reality, an attempt at recovery, a process of reconstruction" (Freud, 1911, p. 70). Later he wrote that the "delusion is found like a patch over the place where originally a rent had appeared in the ego's relation to the external world" (Freud, 1924, p. 151).

Much later Freud (1940) went on to argue that the loss of contact with reality in psychosis was never complete and that a healthy part of the mind continued to exist even in the most severe cases of psychosis. He stated that,

> One learns from patients after their recovery that at the time in some corner of their mind (as they put it) there was a normal person hidden who, like a detached spectator, watched the hubbub of illness go past him. (Freud, 1940, pp. 201–202)

Freud described the co-existence of two psychical attitudes, one which took account of reality and another which under the influence of the instincts detached the ego from reality, and he believed that when the abnormal one gained the upper hand then the situation was ripe for the onset of psychosis.

Bion (1957, p. 56) developed these ideas further by characterising the two coexisting psychical attitudes as the psychotic and non-psychotic parts of the personality. He stated that the psychotic part attacked all aspects of the perceiving ego responsible for the registration of internal and external reality, minutely fragmenting and projecting all aspects of the mind necessary for emotional assessments. The psychotic part's aim was to impose a total withdrawal from reality by smashing up these sense impressions and projecting them into external objects outside the self. These objects then would take on the characteristics of the projections to form "bizarre objects" that would then suffuse and control the projected piece of the personality. This created a diffusely persecuting and terrifying atmosphere, akin to a "nameless dread". In doing so, the psychotic part of the personality prevented the formation of thoughts or attacked the links between different thoughts in an attempt to render the patient mindless.

Nevertheless, contact with reality was never lost due to the continuing existence of a non-psychotic part of the personality functioning in parallel which meant that the psychotic part of the personality could never entirely succeed in cutting itself off from psychic pain (Lucas, 2009).

Steiner (1993) understands psychotic states as arising when ordinary defensive measures fail either under pressure from internal or external factors, resulting in a terrifying anxiety arising out of the threat of total self disintegration. Such is the extreme nature of the threat posed by reality that attacks are mounted against the perceiving mind itself, resulting in a fundamental break between the self and the external world. Steiner argues that in such circumstances of "overwhelming confusion, uncontrolled panic and intense anxiety" (Steiner, 1993, p. 68), the only solution is to turn towards a psychotic organisation, which even if recognised as mad, provides a better alternative to the catastrophic anxiety experienced outside. The psychotic part of the personality relieves the patients' anxieties by providing an omnipotent retreat where these anxieties can be organised into a delusional system where the source of persecution becomes clear. This provides relief from anxiety but at the disabling expense of having to live in a psychotic world. Steiner describes the situation as follows:

> It sometimes appears as if the patient believes that the 'rent' between the ego and reality results from an attack on his mind, leaving a tear through which mental contents will fall out, leaving nothing morethan an empty shell. The psychotic organization is then called in to repair the rent by providing a patch which makes the patient feel more whole and less in danger of disintegrating .... What appeared as a nameless and vague dread becomes converted into a clear-cut delusion of persecution with apparent relief. (Steiner, 1993, p. 66)

Steiner (1993, p. 64) further emphasises the fragility of these psychotic organisations; they are rarely stable as the anxieties which threaten the individual as the organisation begins to break down are usually conspicuous since reality continually tries to assert itself. At the same time, however, the catastrophic nature of these anxieties reinforces the pull and desperate dependence on these organisations in order to avoid a return of the uncontrolled panic associated with imminent annihilation.

Lucas (2009) repeatedly drew our attention to how the psychotic part of the personality could cover up its murderous activity by appearing calm and reasonable and how this had major implications for the ongoing management of these types of cases. In particular, each time we have to make an assessment of a patient with a suggested history of psychosis, Lucas asked us to consider whether we are hearing a straightforward communication from the non-psychotic part or are being invited to accept a rationalisation from the psychotic part.

Clinical material

I am going to describe, based on clinical material and the court records of a patient, the composite case of a young woman who killed her mother. As a successful tennis player she was bright, beautiful, disciplined, mature, and highly regarded among her peers and teammates. The twenty-two-year-old was at the centre of a loving family proudly involved in tennis circles. To everyone her life seemed happy and trouble free. But suddenly something in Ms A changed that led her to kill her mother. Mother and daughter had a mutual love for tennis, and their shared passion meant they were continually together.

> In the summer, Ms. A began to experience a build up of stress that damaged her outlook and led to devastating consequences. Ms. A was deeply affected after breaking up with her boyfriend, her first serious relationship, when she suspected that he had been unfaithful. This relationship started soon after Ms A's grandmother had passed away—the first time she had experienced the loss of a close relative. She began to feel unsure whether she should drop out of university. She began to feel quite pressured while competing in high level tennis matches. She resorted to excessive drinking on nights out with friends and later admitted having suicidal thoughts. She then lost interest in tennis, faked injuries and was pleased when she received text messages saying that training had been called off. Something had changed for Ms A in that her environment was not quite the same.
>
> Her family noticed that she had become quiet and withdrawn, often opting to sit alone in her bedroom and appearing as if she was in another world. But the devastating extent of her so called depressed mood only became clear during an incident at the family home shortly after a Sunday dinner. Ms A coaxed her father into the utility room and attempted to stab him with a kitchen knife. She said that it was in her head to do it: "I was going to kill my dad," she told a psychologist; "I had the knife in my hand, I raised the knife and attempted to stab his neck." Her father asked her why she did it; he told the court: "She said she wanted me to go to heaven. She said I could look after her better there."
>
> The father said that he was in total shock and arranged for her to see the GP the next day, who referred her to a counsellor at an addiction awareness charity. She was diagnosed with depressive disorder that impaired her mental functioning. The GP said that Ms A came to believe that killing one of her parents would resolve her unhappiness by making them her "guardian in heaven". Ms A would later say that that she felt that, "killing someone would settle you down a lot more. I was going to kill someone. I knew it was going to be one of my parents; when you had these thoughts it seemed as if all your problems would go away, that you would be happy, that you could carry on with your life a bit longer."
>
> However, her health was not assessed by a psychiatrist before tragedy struck. Ms A felt the counselling session did not help; she only had one session, and thoughts of killing one of her parents soon began to resurface again.

> Several months after the attempted knifing of her mother, Ms A again harboured thoughts of killing her father. But throughout the day she appeared her usual self, chatting and later playing tennis with friends. However, she felt unable to go through with her intention to kill her father, instead she decided to kill her mother on her return home. She waited outside with her knife—"My heart went fast; I felt powerful"—and as her mother came home and got out her car, Ms A stabbed her mother. She knelt beside her mother, said sorry and considered taking her own life but decided against it. She drove to the neighbour and said, "Mummy is dead."
>
> She initially told the police there had been a burglary at the home, but later the same night, sitting on the edge of a bed in her home, Ms A confessed to the killing of her mother. Before being taken away by the police, Ms A was allowed to speak to her father. "We just lay on the single bed, we just hugged and cuddled each other, we were both crying" he later told the court.

This clinical vignette illustrates many of the psychoanalytic ideas discussed earlier, and although chosen for these reasons, it is nevertheless a typical scenario one commonly comes across in the hospitals and prisons in which we work. In characteristic fashion little information is gained from the patient. In nearly all such cases, the crime is rationalised and made sane to the extent that the incident is turned into a trivial misunderstanding. The patient one is confronted with appears calm and reasonable, expressing her remorse.

The trial

At the trial, conflicting details of Ms A's mental state in the weeks prior to killing her mother were presented. Asked by prosecuting counsel whether the accused was capable of forming rational judgments, the consultant forensic psychiatrist, Dr B, replied, "Yes, she was."

Earlier Dr B had said that Ms A told him she never thought about the consequences of killing her mother. During cross-examination, defence counsel asked if Ms A's behaviour around the time she carried out the stabbing was irrational. He replied: "It's certainly not normal thinking; it's abnormal ... but certainly not indicative of mental illness." The psychiatrist was also asked if it was possible Ms A was developing schizophrenia. "In my opinion there are a number of reasons to be alert to the possibility that Ms A may be developing schizophrenia," he replied. However, he added: "I'm satisfied that at present there are not sufficient features to make a diagnosis of schizophrenia."

Prosecuting Counsel referred to Ms A's behaviour around the time of her grandmother's death, including a loss of interest in tennis, heavy drinking, and suicidal thoughts. Dr B said the "overall picture" of depressive symptoms was not strong enough to make a depressive episode diagnosis. Prosecuting Counsel put it to Dr B that he was "going to the book and seeing what boxes can be ticked". Dr B added: "My view is that she did not meet the criteria for a major depressive episode, even a mild depressive episode, but I accept she did have depressive symptoms." Questioned on Ms A's suicidal thoughts, Dr B added: "One would not diagnose depressive illness on the basis of suicidal thoughts alone." However, the doctor conceded that some sufferers of depression, particularly young people, can mask their condition effectively.

Ms A's father said she "never gave us any bother" until he noticed she had become withdrawn. Her father said he was in the utility room with his daughter examining a leaking tumble dryer when she began sobbing and told him her boyfriend had left her. He said he told his daughter not to worry as she was still a young woman and would find someone else. He said she replied that she did not want anyone else. He added: "I was turning to go out of the garage when I felt a knife come towards my neck." He ran out of the garage door and Ms A was saying that she didn't mean it. He asked her "what's going on?" "She said that she wanted me to go to heaven to look after her and grandmother." The sobbing father said that his daughter's grandmother had died some time before, and Ms A was very close to her. Father said: "I don't want to go to heaven. I want to stay here with you." She said: "I hope you will always be very proud of me." I said that I would always be proud of her.

When asked if he could explain what had happened, he said: "There is no reason at all as to why she would want to kill me. I thought there was something seriously wrong with her. We were very concerned. We didn't know what we were dealing with." He said his wife made an appointment the following day with their family GP, who said their daughter did not need any medication but recommended that she see a counsellor.

He said he and his daughter later drove separately to the appointment, where she spent around an hour and a half with the counsellor whom she only saw once. He said that following the incident in the garage, he found that his daughter had changed and that she increasingly spent more time out of the house, keeping herself to herself and playing music. She would be very snappy at times and very vague in her answers.

Finally, Ms A's father read a letter to the jury which Ms A had written while on remand and wanted to be read at the funeral. It said: "To my special mum, this is just a short note. You have been a great mum. I love you and I will miss you in my life."

Ms A herself denied murdering her mother at their family home. She admitted killing her mother, but her defence team said it was "a very clear case of diminished responsibility". Ms A's barrister said a manslaughter verdict would be the "right, just, and proper thing to do". He said the central question was how a young woman of impeccable character, with everything in the world to live for, came to develop bizarre notions that killing one of her parents would help her to cope with her problems in life. She had stabbed her mother shortly after breaking up with her boyfriend. However the prosecution said the break-up of a relationship was no excuse for murder. In his summing up, a prosecution barrister described Ms A as "brutally selfish" in killing her mother in order to get over whatever upset she had in her life. He said it gave the accused feelings of control and excitement and she had shown little empathy for her victim. The barrister told the jury that although Ms A was a gifted tennis player and a good sportswoman with a good life given to her by a good family, she was a treacherous woman. Beneath her smiling face was a "wicked, planning, manipulative killer" the lawyer said.

Ms A had described the killing to police as an "incident", but the prosecution lawyer said that it wasn't an incident; it was the slaughter of her mother, planned and executed meticulously by her. The prosecution barrister said there was no evidence that the accused was suffering from mild depression, nor that her alleged mental condition had an impact on her understanding, rational judgment or ability to demonstrate self-control, which would provide a defence to the murder charge. He said that Ms A's feeling a bit down, following the break-up with her boyfriend, was not an excuse for murdering someone.

But Ms A's defence barrister said that not once during the trial had the prosecution suggested any motive for murder. He told the jury not to be blinded by expert evidence and asked them: "Do you really need to be a psychiatrist to know that something in this young woman's head was badly wrong?" He said it was not in dispute that the manner of the mother's death was simply horrific, and that her daughter, being in the dock charged with her murder, was perhaps the ultimate tragedy.

He added that Ms A's attempt to stab her father before the shooting was a dreadful spine-chilling incident that was every father's worst possible nightmare. But the defence lawyer said that this incident was the window that sheds light on this whole case; it shows beyond all doubt that she was suffering from deluded thinking and abnormality of mental functioning. He said manslaughter was not a soft option and was not an attempt to avoid Ms A's responsibility for the death of her father, but that her responsibility was diminished by her mental state at the time of the killing.

Applying the ID cluster list

A. **The <u>patient</u> repeatedly perceives <u>others</u> so that they are** accepting and admiring (**affirming**) towards her; even that they treat her as a special (**idealising**) daughter and athlete.

At the other extreme, she sees them as deserting and ignoring **(abandoning)** and rejecting and excluding **(destroying)** her: her boyfriend betrays and leaves her and her grandmother dies.

In her delusion she perceives others as attending to and caring for her in every way (**protecting**): she wants her parents to be in heaven as her eternal guardians.

B. **The patient regularly experiences herself as** insisting on her position (**asserting**): she is convinced that securing a guardian in heaven even by killing is the right thing to do. This implies that she sees herself as special (**idealising**) and behaving as though she knows best (allowing independence).

On the other hand, again at the opposite extreme, it can be inferred that she feels utterly despairing (submitting): unable to tolerate the concrete threats of personal annihilation posed by the loss of such significant figures.

C. **Others, the staff included, regularly perceive the patient as** over relying on and draining (**depending**): she feels devastated when her boyfriend leaves her and her grandmother dies, totally unable to confront the task of mourning and face the prospect of life without them. As a consequence, in her murderous actions and delusion she totally absorbs the separate life of her mother/father guardian in heaven. The latter also reflects qualities of being domineering and imposing (**controlling**) and intimidating and attacking (**destroying**). Finally, others perceive Ms A as running away (**recoiling**) from her daily activities by giving up her university course and tennis;

as well as demonstrating a more radical cutting off contact (**isolating**) through immersion in her delusional world.

D. Others, the staff included, regularly experience themselves as supporting and agreeing and accepting and admiring (**affirming**): **she is** highly regarded by family and friends to the extent of feeling over involved and over sympathetic (reactive idealising), attending to and caring (protecting) and appeasing and complying with (submitting): not wanting to give her a psychiatric diagnosis, thus, treating her as normal; lying in bed with her after the killing of mother.

These latter aspects would be most difficult for others to acknowledge. Nevertheless, it is precisely such collusion with the psychotic part of Ms A's personality—the affirming, reactive, idealising, and submitting elicited under perspective D of the Interpersonal Dynamics cluster list—which represents a profound abandonment and rejection of her non-psychotic capacity to recognise her dependency needs, intense anxieties and continuing potential for violence. Consequently, her terror of being abandoned and destroyed (Perspective A) is reinforced as she is left to herself to contain the uncontainable; and paradoxically her murderously delusional solution is also only intensified.

The transition between perspectives C and D is particularly interesting and crucial: how can staff/others clearly recognise Ms A's dependency, controlling, destroying, and recoiling/isolating characteristics yet respond with such collusion? Even the protecting quality can be maladaptive (protecting her from a diagnosis which acknowledges the reality of her mental illness). The answer, as indicated above, seems to be that standing up to the psychotic part of the personality poses grave risks; even the defence team, whose protecting quality does appear to be in touch with Ms A's needs for treatment rather than prison, does not have to undergo the fraught process of establishing a prolonged relationship with both parts of Ms A's personality which treatment will involve. The defence team, unlike the mental health team, does not risk the intrinsic murderous encounter with the psychotic part of the personality.

Expanded formulation and discussion

Having completed this survey of the ID perspectives, I will try to relate them to one another. Ms A feels people are concerned and caring about her, but they also abandon her: her grandmother died and her boyfriend rejected her. At the same time she feels intensely dependent on her family. She initially feels that she has to run away or isolate herself, then begins to feel a dread that they will abandon her and she will be annihilated. This is the beginning of a vicious circle in that the more she depends on her family, the more she will become weakened; and thus to overcome her feeling of weakness, smallness, and dread, she develops an omnipotent and omniscient idea or delusion that she has to put her parents in heaven in order that they will always look after her. Thus, she has taken control and feels powerful and omnipotent in that she can place her parents in heaven and in that way live happily ever after with no anxiety, convinced that she will be looked after forever.

The psychotic structure is like a delusional world or object into which parts of the self tend to withdraw. It appears to be dominated by an omnipotent, or omniscient, extremely ruthless part of the self which creates the notion that within the delusional object there is complete painlessness but also freedom to indulge in any sadistic activity (Rosenfeld, 1971, pp. 169–178). The destructive impulses within this delusional world sometimes appear as overpoweringly cruel, threatening the rest of the self with death if they assert their power; but more frequently they appear disguised as omnipotent, benevolent or life saving: promising to provide the patient with quick ideal solutions to all her problems. These false promises are designed to make the normal self of the patient dependent on or addicted to her omnipotent self and to lure the normal sane parts—as well as professionals—into this delusional structure in order to imprison them.

Thus psychosis can be considered a two stage process: initially there is a psychic catastrophe, characterised by a **denial or disavowal** of unacceptable reality with a resulting feeling that there is something in the air, an oppressive tension; this is followed by the creation of a substitute reality in the **form of delusions and hallucinations** to make good the damage done, and often with a feeling of relief from the unbearable tension (Freud, 1924).

> Thus her family noticed that she had become quiet and withdrawn, often opting to sit alone in her bedroom and appeared as if she was in another world, the delusional mood.

Freud (1911) emphasised that many of the symptoms of psychosis arose from attempts on the parts of the patient to restore her **damaged ego and to reconstitute a world which had been destroyed**: in other words the delusional formation, which we take to be the pathological product, is in reality an attempt at recovery, a process of reconstruction.

> "She said she wanted me to go to heaven. She said I could look after her better there." The GP said that Ms A came to believe that killing one of her parents would resolve her unhappiness by making them her "guardian in heaven". Ms A would later say that that she felt that "killing someone would settle you down a lot more. I was going to kill someone. I knew it was going to be one of my parents, when you had these thoughts it seemed as if all your problems would go away, that you would be happy; that you could carry on with your life a bit longer."

Freud (1924) also noted the anxiety that accompanied the symptoms of psychosis and suggested that this was due to the hated and denied reality continuing to force itself upon the mind.

> The idea that her parents had to go to heaven to look after her seemed to resurface after her first attempted stabbing of father, but with much more force in that she seemed more determined in order to move into the realm of concrete action and so evacuate the tension of her overwhelming anxieties that she would remain alone and completely vulnerable forever.

Psychotic states arise when ordinary defensive measures fail under massive pressures and anxieties such as severe loss which trigger an imminent threat of annihilation, the only solution to which is to turn to a psychotic organisation which offers relief from the terrible anxiety at the great expense of living in a psychotic world.

> Ms. A was deeply affected after breaking up with her boyfriend, her first serious relationship, when she suspected that he had been unfaithful. This relationship started soon after Ms A's grandmother had passed away—the first time she had experienced the loss of a close relative. She was also unsure whether she should drop out of university and began to feel intensely pressured competing in high level tennis.

Duncan Cartwright (2002), in discussing rage murder, describes how people keep their murderousness concealed and out of sight. By a particular use of projective identification, the self identifies with idealised people who are psychically held "outside" so as to keep them away from the buried and unseen badness or murderousness inside, which he called a "**narcissistic exoskeleton**". Thus it is the projection of idealised goodness outside, with badness internalised and hidden, which commonly induces in the treatment team the belief that the person is not a killer and that she is, in fact, a nice and reasonable woman.

In these concepts of **buried badness or murderousness** there is always a psychically traumatic and indigestible experience to do with loss and death and a failure of symbolisation. Only with a life threatening trigger, displayed as the fear of death, do they enact their murderousness. Thus a patient, provoked by some particular trigger, usually to do with loss and the fear of death with a consequent weakening and complete collapse of his defensive structure, shifts from identification with a previously idealised version of the self to identification with a previously buried bad version of the self. The latter is experienced as an unbearable and intolerable intrusion of the self which threatens survival. Either it can lead to suicide or it is evacuated and projected into a victim who is then experienced as life threatening, and the murderous attack is represented as an attempt to destroy the threat of the bad object which at that point is experienced concretely as the fear of death or annihilation within the victim or, as in the patient described, the preservation of the good object: paradoxically the act of murder is to preserve the good object.

Violence or murder is the acting out of a narrative (Doctor, 2008); it is thus a communication about these patients' belief systems about themselves, about their relationships with others and about their origins. The patient may be communicating a belief that the truth is unbearable and that evasion of the truth is the sole means of surviving and preventing a catastrophe.

In this particular patient the court case exemplified the split between those who felt the patient was too disturbed to know what she was doing and those who were impressed by her calm reasonableness and therefore willing to minimise the patient's disturbance. However, the psychologist for the defence thought she was depressed and/or psychotic and was struck by the "madness" of the situation, whereas the psychiatrist for the prosecution thought she was sane. In this case the jury found the patient to have diminished responsibility and to be not guilty of murder.

Usually the psychotic condition is so bizarre that in the court case and in the mental health setting the prosecution team/staff find it increasingly difficult to think deeply about the problem and are drawn into asking the sort of "standard" psychiatric questions one might ask in such a situation, while the patient returns the compliment by trotting out the "standard line" in patient answers. Patient and professionals can, therefore, become involved in a charade whereby the professionals are pulled in to support the patient's psychotic organisation in its attempt to impersonate sanity. With the individual application of the ID consultation, instead of relying on the standard psychiatric questions and diagnostics, "going to the book and seeing what boxes could be ticked" (a very distant and cut off way of relating to the patient and his problems), a more reflective and dynamic way of considering the issues is encouraged.

Acknowledgement

The author gratefully acknowledges the contributions to this chapter of John Gordon and Gabriel Kirtchuk.

References

Bion, W. R. (1957). Differentiation of the psychotic from the non-psychotic personalities. *International Journal of Psychoanalysis, 38*: 266–275. Reprinted in *Second Thoughts*. London: Heinemann, 1967.

Cartwright, D. (2002). *Psychoanalysis, Violence and Rage-Type Murder: Murdering Minds*. London: Brunner-Routledge.

Darnley, B., Doctor, R., Gordon, J., & Kirtchuk, G. (2011). Psychotic processes in forensic institutions. *Psychoanalytic Psychotherapy, 25*(1): 55–68.

Doctor, R. (2003). *Dangerous Patients: A Psychodynamic Approach to Risk Assessment and Management*. London: Karnac.

Doctor, R. (2008). *Murder: A Psychoanalytic Investigation*. London: Karnac.

Freud, S. (1911a). Psychoanalytic notes on an autobiographic account of a case of paranoia (Dementia Paranoides). In: J. Stachey (Ed. & Trans.), *The Standard Edition of the Complete Psychological Works of Sigmund Freud* (Vol. 12) (pp. 3–82). London: Hogarth Press.

Freud, S. (1924). Neurosis and psychosis. In: J. Stachey (Ed. & Trans.), *The Standard Edition of the Complete Psychological Works of Sigmund Freud* (Vol. 19) (pp. 149–157). London: Hogarth Press.

Freud, S. (1940). An outline of psychoanalysis. In: J. Stachey (Ed. & Trans.), *The Standard Edition of the Complete Psychological Works of Sigmund Freud* (Vol. 23) (pp. 141–207). London: Hogarth Press.

Lucas, R. (2009). *The Psychotic Wavelength: A Psychoanalytic Perspective for Psychiatry*. London: Routledge.

Rosenfeld, H. (1971). A clinical approach to the psychoanalytic theory of the life and death instincts: an investigation into the aggressive aspects of narcissism. *International Journal of Psychoanalysis, 52*: 169–178.

Steiner, J. (1993). *Psychic Retreats: Pathological Organisations in Psychotic, Neurotic and Borderline Patients*. London: Routledge.

CHAPTER FIVE

Elucidating triggers to violence and improving risk assessment using the ID consultation: an in-depth case study approach

Amber Fossey, David Reiss, and Gabriel Kirtchuk

Introduction

Assessing risk of recidivism is a critical component of treatment in secure mental health services. It is not enough to treat mental illness and assume risk is ameliorated as a result. In order to implement effective risk management plans and prevent violence, mental health professionals must be alert to dynamic interpersonal factors, which may recur in a patient's circumstances and cause risk to subsequently increase.

The status quo in clinical risk assessment is that we look at historical risk events but do not consider lifelong relational triggers. Examination of historical risk factors has long been recognised as essential in the commonly used structured professional judgement tool, the HCR-20, with the "H" representing "Historical" (Webster, Douglas, Eaves, & Hart, 1997). What is less widely adopted is a multidisciplinary examination of interpersonal patterns in a patient's personal history and in their current relationships, including those within the treatment setting. To the authors this seems a curious omission, given both the specific presence of a disordered interpersonal exchange between any violent offender and his/her victim and the more general, often starkly apparent, interpersonal problems which characterise forensic mental health patients.

Various models of causality have been proposed to describe the relationship between risk factors and violence. Causal dynamic risk factors can be categorised as traits, which are chronic and recurring, such as psychosis and drug use, or an acute single event such as extreme arousal. Studies have demonstrated that it is quite possible to explore the narrative of a violent incident and deduce from it an apparent trigger such as reaction to insult, grudge, fear of attack or provocation by victim. However, this could be an over-simplification in that there might be deeper processes at work between offender and victim which have precipitated violence. Freestone (2014) explored whether triggers to violence could be detected retrospectively using a cohort of 514 male and female prisoners who had committed violent index offences. Police National Computer records revealed any subsequent convictions for violence over a seven year follow-up period. The study elicited sixteen triggers from subject interviews ranging from psychosis, intoxication, and argument to the less tangible humiliation or threatened loss. The authors concluded that most acute risk factors do not predict future violence, except psychosis and alcohol intoxication. The identification of these factors does not however reveal underlying primitive compulsions to act violently. It may be that in psychosis, for example, maladaptive defences are more disturbed than in a non-psychotic individual. Similarly, disinhibition resulting from alcohol or drug intoxication may lead to a lower threshold for distorted cognitions to be acted on, such as a paranoid belief others are always attacking.

Triggers were further explored and categorised by McMurran (2012). This study examined violence explicitly in the context of alcohol intoxication with a smaller cohort of young male offenders and used thematic analysis of perpetrators' verbal accounts to extract sixteen types of trigger. These were then assimilated into six common themes or categories, including being offended, distress, an opportunity for material gain, and perception of threat. Such categories incorporated practical incentives for violence alongside emotional drivers such as a need to offset the pain of being insulted. All categories could be said to be instrumental in some regard, except "wanting a fight", which appears a spurious reason perhaps obscuring an unconscious drive with its own purpose. McMurran found, at least with alcohol on board, that reactive aggression was most common and was often confounded by hypermasculine values and sensitivity to disrespect. These defences may be survival strategies resulting from disturbed early life experiences and entail a hostile attribution bias. Such underlying features may also be common to Freestones stable trait risk factors such as drug use and impulsivity. McMurran's aim was to use the risk themes identified in his study to devise appropriate individual level interventions so that an offender can recognise potential provocations and learn to cognitively reappraise the situation before resorting to violence. It could be speculated that alcohol as a risk factor is merely a catalyst for the disinhibition of unconscious relationship scenarios and associated affects which, precisely because they operate out of awareness, would not be elicited at a later date by offender interview.

A sample of domestic violence perpetrators was examined by Ross and Babcock (2009). Ross and Babcock proposed that domestic violence differed in its function depending on the personality disorder subtype of the offender. They found that men with emotionally unstable, borderline type personalities appeared to use violence reactively in response to perceived provocation, and that this correlated to previous typologies of "impulsive" or "pathologically dependent" batterers. This profile is also similar to those with a preoccupied attachment style whose violence functioned as an expressive response to abandonment fears. Ross and Babcock contrasted this with proactive violence in the absence of anger by antisocial personality disordered offenders, akin to instrumental, cold-blooded or premeditated violence. This typology further delineated specific types of trigger depending on whether the violence was reactive or proactive, such as wives making a demand or being defiant triggering proactive violence, or a partner threatening to leave triggering reactive violence. It is an integral diagnostic feature of personality disorder that interpersonal dynamics are disturbed and damaging relationship patterns from early family experiences are repeated in work, social and intimate domains in adulthood. Application of ID tools in cases where a patient has a personality disorder and a history of violence can improve risk assessment and risk management by exploring these disturbed patterns of relating in more detail, as will be demonstrated in the case study.

It is the authors' proposition that exploring interpersonal aspects of a patient's early life and later relationships, in addition to an inspection of events preceding violence, can greatly enhance the deduction of triggers to violence and improve risk assessment (Reiss & Kirtchuk, 2009). We all tend to repeat unconscious patterns of relating to others in intimate relationships, whether adaptive or self-defeating, so it is understandable that offenders too are likely to repeat their patterns of violence irrespective of external circumstance. Application of an Interpersonal Dynamics (ID) consultation within rehabilitative units and amongst multidisciplinary teams can serve to promote recognition of early warning signs of violence and unify therapeutic approaches.

The ID consultation has been established by Kirtchuk and colleagues (2013) as a development of the Operationalized Psychodynamic Diagnostics (OPD) approach described by Stasch (2004). It is able to reveal the underlying dynamics of a patient's interactions in a way that can be comprehended and contributed to by all multidisciplinary team members, utilising the subjective experience of both staff and patient as they relate to each other.

The basic procedure, as described by Kirtchuk and colleagues (2013), is to conceptualise four perspectives of the patients core relationship patterns by clarifying (A) how the patient characteristically perceives the other; (B) how the patient responsively experiences himself; (C) how others (including staff members) usually perceive the patient; and (D) how others/staff experience themselves in their interactions with the patient. The perspectives concern the transference–countertransference configurations enacted between patient and staff, as experienced in the care setting. These are elicited via a multidisciplinary staff team meeting with an ID facilitator. It is important that as many staff perspectives as possible are represented in the assessment because patients treat individual members of a team in very different ways. If certain staff are not present in the ID consultation, then valuable information about risk can be missed as the polarity of views may go unrecognised.

Firstly in the meeting there is a presentation of the case history with particular attention to the nature and quality of significant relationships between the patient and others throughout their life. The reasons for referral are discussed, and the status of current relationships with staff is explored. Staff are then asked to select numbered items between one and thirty-two from an ID cluster sheet by identifying which items most closely correspond to each of the four interpersonal perspectives A–D. The interactions described by the ID cluster tool are categorised as "active" (items one to sixteen) or "reactive" (items seventeen to thirty-two). Active interactions focus on how the "self" (patient or staff) in a relationship believes "others" are treating him, and reactive interactions elicit the "self's" responses to such treatment. For example, a patient who said, "The staff let me have extra leave because I'm their favourite" would be evidence supporting item A-5: "The patient repeatedly perceives others as treating him as special" (active). Usually a maximum of four items are chosen for each perspective A–D based on having the most cogent evidence. On the basis of the selected items, the team then attempts to make a dynamic formulation by linking A–B–C–D–A, for example, "The patient repeatedly perceives others as ..., and in response, the patient experiences himself as ... continuing on, others repeatedly perceive the patient as ... and in response experience themselves as ..." D can then be linked back to A, and a vicious circle of relating to others is revealed. This formulation of the patient's patterns of current relationships can be mapped back onto their early relationships by means of a subsequent, expanded formulation. Once the core dynamics are identified, it becomes possible to link past experiences in the patient's life with unwitting repetitions of those past patterns between patient and staff.

We offer a case study below to demonstrate how the application of an ID perspective can help to identify violent triggers. (The case is fictitious, based on an amalgam of previous clinical experience.)

For the purposes of this study we will label events temporally immediate to violence as "triggers". We acknowledge the influence of counterfactual thinking, whereby it is human nature to attribute more causal weight to events which occur most proximal to an outcome, and do not wish to underestimate the power of sub-acute interpersonal factors in the days or weeks before; rather, that is not the focus of our discussion.

Case study: the bowls, the knife, and the special boy

Mr Y is a middle aged white British male detained on a medium secure rehabilitation ward in a forensic psychiatric hospital. His index offence occurred some years earlier when he attempted to murder his wife by stabbing her in the back. He was an only child and recalls his mother telling him that he ripped her insides apart during childbirth. His mother had a son out of wedlock before Mr Y whom she was forced to give up for adoption. Mr Y explains this as the cause of her possessive control over him. He recalled the relationship with his mother as a difficult one. He said his mother manipulated him to get what she wanted and has made his life a misery; "My mother emotionally blackmailed me" and "My mother gave me a terrible life." According to Mr Y after his birth his mother suffered postnatal depression which persisted into long term depression and required ECT. He felt he cared for his mother: "I helped my mother a lot."

Mr Y said he felt unloved by his father, who ran a bakery. He recounts that his parents gave him money but devoted all their time to the business, neglecting to spend time with him or show him any affection. He recalls his childhood as very unhappy. Mr Y's recollection of his childhood suggested high expressed emotion within his family. For example, there was a big row when he asked to go out for an evening as an adolescent, his mother begged him to stay and he subsequently submitted.

Mr Y left school at sixteen without qualifications. He soon married, had one child, a son, and worked in a supermarket stacking shelves during his twenties. During this period he developed depression, which became chronic over the course of the next thirty years. There is a suggestion that he drank alcohol heavily, but he never became dependent. A few months prior to the index offence, he stopped the medication he had taken for many years because the pharmacy ran out of stock, and he decided he didn't want to take any more medication. He suffered physical and mental withdrawal, lost his job and his mood spiraled down. He heard voices and felt anxious and confused. The day before the index offence he went to his GP to report a dream of murdering his wife. He recalled that he requested immediate psychiatric help but felt dismissed by his GP, despite being given new tablets and urgently referred to the community mental health team. The next day, by his account, his wife began berating him for not finding a new job before leaving the room and walking to the kitchen, at which point he felt sudden rage. Mr Y followed her, grabbed a kitchen knife and stabbed her multiple times from behind. He had no prior history of domestic violence or criminal offending. On later questioning, Mr Y said, "I tried to kill her and myself because I wanted to be with her forever."

In prison after the offence, Mr Y engaged in numerous episodes of self-harm including burns and wounds to his chest. After some months in prison he was transferred to hospital. He responded well to antipsychotic and antidepressant medication. He was diagnosed with late onset schizophrenia and depression, the differential diagnosis being psychotic depression. He has also been described as having borderline and narcissistic personality traits. There have been concerns that his cognitive abilities, in particular memory, have been declining, although not to a level of dementia. At his last mental health tribunal he received a deferred conditional discharge pending placement at a twenty-four hour staffed hostel. He has a non-contact order applicable to his wife, from whom he is now divorced, and an exclusion zone applied by the Ministry of Justice covering an entire borough where his ex-wife and extended family live.

A referral for an ID consultation was instigated due to several concerns raised by the treating team. The social worker complained that she had found a perfect hostel but that Mr Y was being obstructive towards the placement. She said there had been a repeating pattern of him trying to sabotage discharge. Subsequently, Mr Y approved a hostel which he then held in high regard compared to the hospital. He said hostel staff treated him wonderfully, attended to all his needs, and that he could not wait to leave the hospital.

The occupational therapist (OT) was vexed that Mr Y broke a promise about spending money on bowls equipment. They had visited a sports shop together as Mr Y said he wanted to start playing bowls now that he was approaching discharge. Historically Mr Y had difficulty managing his money; hence the OT had agreed a budget with him. The OT was later telephoned by an elderly in-law of Mr Y to complain he had harassed her into lending him money for more bowls. The OT felt Mr Y had been manipulative and exploitative. In addition he had accrued a debt to the sports shop by upgrading several of his purchases, which the OT felt was another deceit. This pattern was repeated for several weeks. Staff were frustrated with his overspending, exasperated with his apparent irresponsibility and refused to release more money. Mr Y seemed indignant and demanding, and he accused staff of cruelty and neglecting his needs.

High expressed emotions were evident in ward rounds, such as staff raising their voices at Mr Y for his behaviour as though "telling him off" or "nagging". Mr Y would react badly and shout, "Why are you always like this to me? You always tell me what to do! I don't like it." He would also complain that the social worker never returned his calls and no one helped him with his problems: "The staff aren't doing anything about it, the way they treat me hurts me a lot." In contrast, he tended to favour individual staff and praised them highly: "My primary nurse is really good and helps me." He also thought he was a caring figure to his peers: "I help my friends here a lot."

Some members of the team described Mr Y's appearance and manner as "smug and haughty" and that he dressed as though he were "a

> distinguished gentleman in designer clothes", when actually they felt he was quite frail and vulnerable.
>
> As he imminently approached discharge, a ward nurse saw Mr Y having lunch with his ex-wife in a local café despite his non-contact order. Mr Y told staff that his ex-wife had approached him during unescorted leave and asked him to share coffee with her; hence he felt justified he had not breached any rules.

An ID consultation was held with a psychotherapist and the multidisciplinary team. Here a brief interpersonal dynamics formulation for the case is offered.

Time and again Mr Y experiences others as bad objects who patronise him (A8), reject (A14) or ignore (A16) him. In contrast, he tends also to think others are supportive (A3) or treat him as special (A5).

Consequently, he takes a hurt and indignant stance (B27, B28) and reacts assertively by behaving as though he knows best (B2) or even attacking the other (B13). As he thinks others treat him as special, so too does he see himself doing the same (B5).

It is interesting how others repeatedly recognise Mr Y's indignant reproaches as oppositional defiance (C17) and even manipulation (C10). Although often underestimated in this case, staff also see him as intimidating and attacking (C13).

An inevitable outcome of staff seeing the patient as all bad is that they show disgust (D30) and then protect themselves by rejection (D14) or ignoring him (D16), that is, they take flight. In contrast, they often find themselves protecting him (D8).

Not surprisingly, while the staff find themselves taking flight, the patient senses this rejection (A14) and ignoring (A16), and this reinforces his perspective that the world abandons him. He is able also however to recognise the opposing action of protection, as though others treat him as special (A5). It is striking that staffs' views of their own behaviour is quite similar to how he sees them.

After making a basic formulation, we then expand it. In this case we will be using psychodynamic theory, but other approaches could be used.

Mr Y's perception of staff as rejecting or patronising could be seen as an unconscious replication of his feelings towards his parents, a transference re-enactment. His feelings of being patronised and rejected as a child triggered his attempts to assert his rights and independence as an adult, which he continues to do with others now by behaving as though he knows best or by the ultimate seeking of attention, using attack.

The high expressed emotion and disturbed attachments of Mr Y's family group are also re-enacted within the surrogate family of the ward in an echo of his earlier life troubles. We can see a recurring split in the interpersonal dynamics between idealisation of both subject and object and destruction by attack or rejection.

Protection is a dominant cluster in this case. Mr Y perceives and induces protection from others on an axis from controlling to idealising: from the possessive control of his mother to the idealisation of hostel staff. The attempted murder of his wife could be seen as his attempt at ultimate control and total possession because he feared her rejection, highlighted by his comment, "I tried to kill her and myself because I wanted to be with her forever." Therefore, the attempted murder can be seen as a defence against rejection, and rejection is likely to be a definitive trigger for violence in this case.

There is a sense that Mr Y is weak and vulnerable and that his risk is not real. Before the index offence, Mr Y presented his attacking thoughts in a dream, leading his GP to view his potential for risk as surreal and vastly underestimate his attacking capability. Despite years in hospital his diagnosis is vague, staff see him as meek, and "attacking" (C13) was the very last factor to be raised in his ID consultation. His team admitted to minimising or even ignoring his risk behaviour (such as meeting his wife for coffee), perhaps as a defence against the unspoken group anxiety that the patient could seriously jeopardise his discharge or attack again.

The above interpersonal formulation allows for a pause for thought as Mr Y approaches a critical point in his care pathway of discharge to the community after five years in hospital. It allows staff to revisit his HCR-20 risk assessment with an enlightened perspective regarding triggers of risk scenarios, protective factors, and monitoring considerations. It draws attention to a possible bias of underestimating risk and highlights the importance of family work in the community to minimise the risk of Mr Y and his ex-wife repeating past dysfunctional patterns of relating to each other and to professional third parties.

Conclusion and discussion

The use of the ID consultation in the case of My Y identified his entrenched and maladaptive ways of relating to others, as well as his unconscious defences which trigger complementary maladaptive responses from others. In the case of the index offence his defence of attack reached such intensity as to trigger the near fatal stabbing of his wife. We can also conclude from the ID consultation that perceived rejection is a potential trigger for Mr Y's violence. It was therefore formulated that discharge from hospital should be carefully managed and require close monitoring and supervision as the discharge itself could be perceived as a rejection by Mr Y. In addition, it was identified that others have a tendency to perceive Mr Y as benign and to underestimate his risk, which could allow boundary breaches to go unrecognised as staff turn "a blind eye".

The ID consultation is a useful tool for the identification of boundary breaches. In general, major breaches of staff-patient boundaries, such as inappropriate sexual relationships, occur rarely. However, subtle boundary breaches are much more common, particularly with inexperienced staff. Examples include a patient extracting personal information from staff or currying small favours. Such minor breaches often go undetected and become normalised, while the multidisciplinary approach of an ID consultation can highlight the different relationships staff can have with one patient. When dynamics are revealed, staff can explore how they may modify or address the patient's needs to avoid repetition of highly dysfunctional patterns. The ID method encourages staff to adapt their approach rather than challenging or confronting the patient to change his behaviour. It also encourages an objective view of treatment and risk management by removing distracting and dysfunctional interference. It promotes realistic progress in terms of the recovery model approach by supporting the patient's true strengths and avoiding false investment into idealised pseudo-strengths. These modifications can incorporated into the patient's care plan. By integrating an ID consultation into the risk assessment, the latter becomes improved and a stronger risk management plan can be enforced. The ID formulation should be utilised in conjunction with an HCR-20 risk assessment and care plan.

The significance of neonatal life adversity on the developing brain has been explored by Gerhardt (2004). Gerhardt describes the critical neurophysiological sequelae which correlate directly with maladaptive social, behavioural, and emotional performance in later life. For example, chronic stress as a baby can cause over production of cortisol and modulation of other neurotransmitter levels such as serotonin. Low serotonin has been linked to impulsivity and aggression in adulthood. Gerhardt's' point is illustrated in our case above. Factors relevant to index offences, which are elicited by the ID consultation, can be traced back to emotional dysregulation between parent and child in earlier life due to maternal mental ill health, loss, or separation.

ID as a multidisciplinary tool utilises vital, but often unrecognised information to help teams understand maladaptive patterns in patients' core relationships. Not only are these patterns repeated in a broad spectrum across time, place, and person, but they can also be seen in pivotal flashpoints in a patients' history, such as in the circumstances of an index offence.

Newly revealed dynamic risk factors can then be incorporated into the HCR-20 as additional factors. Second, knowledge of the dynamic risk pattern can be useful when generating likely future risk scenarios. Third, insight into how the patient commonly relates to others can guide practical risk management plans, for example, recommendations that the patient should be assessed by staff who represent both sides of a split if the patient tends to polarise opinions.

It is the authors hope that we have demonstrated using case discussion how ID consultations can identify dysfunctional interpersonal relationships and triggers for historical violence, and how identification of such factors can be used to predict violence in similar circumstances in the future. The use of ID thereby facilitates a deeper and more holistic approach to risk assessment and management within secure hospital settings.

Acknowledgement

With thanks to John Gordon and Beate Schumacher.

References

Freestone, M. (2016). *Acute Risk Factors and Triggers for Violence. Criminal Justice and Behavior* (in press).

Gerhardt, S. (2004). *Why Love Matters: How Affection Shapes a Baby's Brain.* London and New York, NY: Routledge.

Kirtchuk, G., Gordon, J., McAllister, M., & Reiss, D. (2013). *Interpersonal Dynamics Consultation—a Manual for Clinicians*. Raleigh, NC: lulu.com.

McMurran, M., Hoyte, H., & Jinks, M. (2012). Triggers for alcohol-related violence in young male offenders. *Legal and Criminal Psychology, 17*: 307–321.

Reiss, D., & Kirtchuk, G. (2009). Interpersonal dynamics and multidisciplinary teamwork. *Advances in Psychiatric Treatment, 15*: 462–469.

Ross, J., & Babcock, J. (2009). Proactive and reactive violence among intimate partner violent men diagnosed with antisocial and borderline personality disorder. *Journal of Family Violence, 24*: 607–617.

Stasch, M. (2004). Interpersonal diagnosis, treatment-focus and clinical implementation based on OPD-axis II. 35th Annual Meeting of the Society for Psychotherapeutic Research, Rome.

Webster, C., Douglas, K., Eaves, D., & Hart, S. (1997). *HCR-20: Assessing Risk for Violence, Version 2*. British Columbia: Mental Health, Law and Policy Institute.

CHAPTER SIX

Working with partner agencies to prevent the abuse and homicide of children

Richard Church, Gabriel Kirtchuk, and David Reiss

> *"I was battered and brutalised my whole childhood—I turned into an orc"*
>
> —Patient in a secure psychiatric ward

Introduction

Any clinician who has experience of working therapeutically with individuals in secure settings will be abundantly aware of the extremely high levels of childhood abuse and neglect in that population. Childhood maltreatment has become a universally accepted risk factor for a trajectory into later antisocial behaviour; strong face validity and evidence from a range of scientific disciplines including population cohort studies, social and psychological sciences, neurodevelopmental research, and gene–environment interaction studies all support what is sometimes referred to as a "cycle of violence". For a multitude of different reasons, it is clear that children who are physically abused by violent parents are more likely to grow up to be violent adults than those children who are not abused.

Child protection services are called upon to intervene in the best interests of children in a challenging and often chaotic multigenerational, multifactorial and multiagency context. It is commonly observed that some cases appear to be particularly and peculiarly problematic, with a lack of objectivity descending like dense fog around the professionals involved, obscuring risks or leading to substantial differences in opinions between professionals. Such difficulties can potentially stall or subvert the primary task of accurate identification and assessment of child safeguarding risks and the delivery of effective child protection.

This chapter describes the context, principles, and clinical significance of child protection, some of the obstacles to effective child safeguarding, and potential benefits that may be gained from consultation approaches informed by psychotherapy to help identify risks and enhance effective multiagency work. The use of a structured approach for consultation with partner agencies is described to help identify dysfunction and highlight risks in a multiagency context.

The significance of child maltreatment

It should come as no surprise that a childhood history of maltreatment is a standard item in many structured risk assessments as a predictor of future violence. The Structured Assessment of Violence Risk in Youth (SAVRY, Borum, Bartel, & Forth, 2015), a "structured professional judgement" kind of risk assessment, states that having a history of victimisation by physical abuse or maltreatment is associated with an increased risk of violence in youth via mechanisms which include exposure to individuals who model violence and who reinforce or reward violent behaviour.

Childhood maltreatment is also included in the Historical Clinical Risk 20 (HCR-20, Webster, 1997) risk assessment of violence under the factor "H8 Early Maladjustment", citing the work of Smith and Thornberry (1995) which identified a dose-sensitive proportionality between the severity of childhood maltreatment and the seriousness of later antisocial behaviour. Safeguarding and protection of children from abuse should therefore be considered to represent a significant intervention in the prevention of violent behaviour at a population level.

At the level of our individual patients, a history of childhood abuse takes a different, clinical significance. A psychotic patient in an acute secure psychiatric setting once said to me, "I was battered and brutalised my whole childhood—I turned into an orc." These stark words from a "raving lunatic" were filled with deep, painful insight and devastating lucidity. He described a history of sustained domestic violence and severe physical abuse towards him and other members of his family that could not be undone, and he clearly identified this as contributing to his current difficulties with a degree of resignation and realism.

Anecdotally, the grievance of this patient and most others that have shared such histories with me was not that social services had interfered unnecessarily in their lives, but rather that "nobody" had stepped in to protect them from the violence they had endured. Interestingly, while working in a high secure psychiatric hospital I learned of cases where a newly appointed social worker had actively followed up disclosures of past abuse that had previously been dropped or overlooked. Her fresh vigour and determination to engage the local police force resulted in successful convictions of perpetrators of serious physical and sexual abuse, sometimes over ten years after the abuse had taken place. The disclosures by psychiatric patients had finally been taken seriously, and the conviction of past abusers contributed to improved therapeutic engagement and patient recovery. Clinicians working directly with individuals in prison or in secure psychiatric settings should be particularly tuned to a history of childhood maltreatment and be equipped with the resources to manage this.

However, not only is child safeguarding important in the prevention of future violence and the therapeutic understanding of our patients—it is of course a very basic principle, enshrined in the United Nations Convention on the Rights of the Child (UNCRC), in Article 19 Protection from all forms of violence and Article 6 Survival and development (UNCRC, 1990). The principle of protecting children from abuse applies to all individuals at all times; clinicians with adult patients should not overlook any potential risks to their patients' children or any children that their patients may have contact with. Despite widespread global support for principles of child safeguarding, the delivery of child protection services varies enormously across the world, with serious failing noted even in well resourced countries. In the UK, clinicians will be familiar with the very high profile achieved by the child safeguarding agenda and documents such as Working Together to Safeguard Children (Department for Education, 2015). Many may have grown weary of yearly, institutionalised mandatory safeguarding training. Nevertheless, despite this high profile and training, we continue to observe repeated serious failures to protect children, sometimes with fatal consequences.

Homicide statistics for England and Wales in the year 2013/2014 (Office for National Statistics, 2015) state that fifty per cent of all victims of homicide aged under sixteen years (twenty-three victims) were killed by their parent or step-parent. A very small number of these cases ever gain media coverage, but when a case does the coverage is often sensationalist and generates a high level of public outrage. A common theme in the press is often the search for someone or somewhere to lay blame, such as a chief executive of children's social services, senior leaders in the police force, or individual social workers, doctors, or teachers. The deaths of Victoria Climbie in 2000 (Department of Health, 2003), Peter Connelly in 2007 (Haringey LSCB, 2009), and Daniel Pelka in 2012 (Local Government Information Unit/Children's Services Network, 2013) are examples of where horrific abuse and torture were somehow overlooked until after the child's death, despite a large number of experienced professionals being involved in the child's life. In the words of BBC reporter Mark Easton (Easton, 2013), Daniel Pelka was "tortured and killed, apparently hidden in full public view". His uncomfortable opinion is that tragic events of this sort were likely to repeat themselves, which indeed is supported by the recent homicide figures of children killed by their parents and carers.

Another uncomfortable emerging view is that these failures may not have been prevented by simply having more resources. The existing pressures on services, including staff shortages and large caseloads, are well recognised and may be exacerbated with further cuts to the public sector; however, these may not be sufficient to explain certain instances of failure to protect children. Similarly, the need for effective case management and supervision structures, as well as the crucial importance of learning from past Serious Case Reviews, have been identified with consequent important changes in practice. Nevertheless, significant failures of safeguarding continue.

A different aspect of safeguarding that has gained significant recent media attention in the UK is the sexual exploitation of teenage girls. Recently, historical abuse perpetrated by high profile individuals including politicians and media celebrities has been highlighted. Operation Yewtree is the name of a British police investigation that was originally set up to investigate allegations of past sexual abuse by the now deceased celebrity Jimmy Savile, who appears to have been a particularly prolific sexual offender against young girls aged between thirteen and sixteen years of age (Gray & Watt, 2013). The public horror at this case is matched by horror at the recent convictions in England for large-scale organised sexual exploitation of teenage girls by groups of men in Rotherham, Rochdale, and Oxfordshire that was somehow previously overlooked or unrecognised.

The reasons for each of these failures of safeguarding differs from one case to another, and each deserves its own thorough investigation and for "lessons to be learnt" and shared. A common theme relevant to this chapter and this book may be that the task of safeguarding children depends on different agencies such as police, social services, education, and health working together more effectively, while at the same time preparing and supporting professionals for the interpersonal challenges raised by the clinical reality of undertaking front line child safeguarding work.

The multiagency landscape

The diagram below (Figure 1) attempts to summarise some of the children's services in existence. Each of these usually has its own particular professional culture, disciplines, language, training, structure, protocols, and information technology systems.

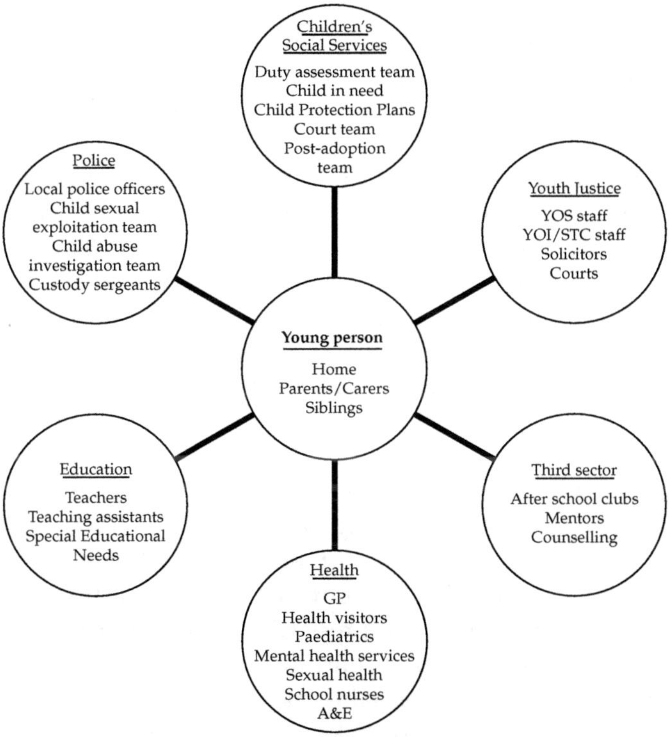

Figure 1. The multiagency landscape of children's services.

Mental health professionals can provide consultation and clinical input to these partner agencies in a variety of ways. Some mental health services are commissioned directly by the agency, and clinicians may be co-located with that agency; in other instances mental health teams may work in parallel in the community, perhaps with a Service Level Agreement or protocol. Sometimes psychotherapists may be commissioned individually to provide reflective staff supervision. In each of these situations, it is imperative to have a clear mutual understanding of the roles and responsibilities undertaken; to fail to do this will be to inevitably add to the chaos that already exists in a challenging context.

In terms of statutory frameworks in England and Wales, the Care Programme Approach (CPA) in adult mental health services provides a central framework for multiagency clinical review, risk assessment, and care planning led by mental health. In children's mental health services CPA is far less commonly used, and statutory planning frameworks are most likely to be led by children's social services (Child in Need and Child Protection Plans), youth offending services (Youth Rehabilitation Orders), or education (Education Health and Care Plans). The ideal of collaborative multiagency work is achieved to varying degrees via these structures.

It should be noted that at a time of decreasing public funds, the number of referrals to child protection services has been steadily increasing over the last few years. There were 657,800 referrals to children's social care in England in 2013–2014, an increase of 10.8% compared to the previous year, and 142,500 section 47 enquiries (detailed child protection investigations) carried out in 2013–2014, an increase of 12.1% on the previous year (Department for Education, 2014).

Youth justice figures indicate an apparently decreasing community need: in 2013/2014 there were 33,902 young people sentenced in England and Wales, representing a fall of twenty-three per cent on the previous year. However, there were 41,569 young people who received a substantive outcome (an out of court or court disposal) in England and Wales in 2013/2014, which only reduced by sixteen per cent from 2012/2013. This indicates that a significant proportion of young people in conflict with the law received an out of court disposal and came into youth justice services under more informal terms (Ministry of Justice and Youth Justice Board for England and Wales, 2015). One may hypothesise that increasing numbers of young people may be being managed via the welfare route of children's social services rather than youth justice.

These figures present the scale of potential opportunities for development of therapeutic multiagency intervention, which is supported by the latest Working Together safeguarding guidance (Department for Education, 2015). Indeed, the national trend in Youth Offending Services and Children's Social Services appears to be moving decidedly towards increasing integration of mental health services and the development of psychologically and psychotherapeutically informed interventions.

A starting point might be to consider what a "child-friendly" children's service might look like. Aspects such as the large number of different social workers that can become involved, high staff turnover, and the number of different professionals and agencies that interact with children have been identified as being problematic for young people. The difficulties are perhaps most stark for those children who have progressed though different children's social work teams and are eventually looked after by their local authority with a general tendency towards repeated changes of placement and a potentially counter-therapeutic lack of stability for the child.

If psychological and psychotherapeutic expertise can be brought to bear on some of these structures and practices, there is scope for improved clinical outcomes, improved staff morale and financial savings by avoiding costly out of borough placements and costs of agency staff.

Interpersonal challenges in child protection

Sound structural and operational aspects of our services are a vital necessity. However, there is another aspect that is central to the core task of service delivery which is often overlooked, learnt "on the job", and seldom taught effectively: how to manage the face-to-face interpersonal challenges of working with complex patients and multidisciplinary teams. I learnt a great deal about physiology and pharmacology at medical school, but I was utterly unprepared for my first patient interaction on my very first day as a junior psychiatrist:

> A tall, muscular patient cornered me in the ward near the locked exit and asked, "Doctor, can I go to the shop to buy cigarettes?", gesturing towards the door. A simple question, but I had no idea how to answer. I was immediately under intense pressure and not inconsiderable threat. It would have been simple for me to just open the door to let him go out—but I felt very uneasy about that. With some alarm at the manner of the

> patient's request, and considerable embarrassment at being clueless around how to answer him, I retreated to the nursing station, and with even further crushing embarrassment I called the Specialist Registrar for advice. What the heck was going on? Medical school had not prepared me for this.

Nobody had warned me that this patient would target me and try to intimidate me as the new, naive but well-meaning junior doctor. The emotional and interpersonal demands I experienced working with that patient were a brand new experience, and with the support of the multidisciplinary team I learnt a great deal.

An exploration of the emotional demands on social workers by Ferguson (2005) calls for the:

> Recognition of the complexities of service users, especially the challenges of working with resistant and often hostile "involuntary clients" and the impact of violence and other health, safety and contamination fears on the capacities of workers and professional networks to protect children. (Ferguson, 2005, p. 781)

Essentially, the pressures of hostile clients and threats of violence that he describes in social work are identical to the interpersonal challenges that are routinely experienced by staff in mental health services, particularly in secure or forensic mental health settings.

There appears to be an interesting overlap between child protection and forensic mental health. The process of safeguarding children involves multiple steps including the identification of risk; conscious appraisal of the nature and severity of the risk; commitment to formulating a written record of the risk; sharing this with relevant agencies; and implementation/delivery of a management plan. Some Serious Case Reviews appear to indicate difficulties with the first few steps, the identification and conscious appraisal of risk. A core role of psychotherapeutically informed consultation to partner agencies can therefore be to explore mechanisms by which safeguarding risks may sometimes be obscured or overlooked, including the following described below.

The sheer horror of child abuse

It has been said that the clinician's ability to detect child abuse is proportional to their ability to conceive it. The horror of a parent or carer actually torturing and killing their child, as was the case with Daniel Pelka, can be so extreme as to be "unthinkable" to clinicians. Indeed, teachers were informed by the "manipulative mother" that Daniel Pelka had a rare genetic disease and should not be fed at school, despite being emaciated and being seen foraging for food in bins. Teachers more readily believed in the presence of a fictitious genetic condition than in such brutal, sustained abuse by his mother who had reportedly locked him in a room, beaten him, starved him, force-fed him salt, and tortured him by putting his head underwater (Local Government Information Unit/Children's Services Network, 2013; Easton, 2013). Indeed, the thought that the parent or carer in front of us may actually present a risk of deliberate harm to their child goes completely against our general cultural assumptions that parents always love, care for, and seek the best for their children.

Parents and carers locating the problem in the child

The task of child protection can be subverted by parents identifying an aspect of the child's health or behaviour as the source of pervasive difficulties for the family and even their own personal problems, often seeking diagnoses or further investigations for the child. This can be associated with fabricated or induced illness and presentation at multiple clinics or professionals.

Attack from parents and carers towards staff

Attack and intimidation from parents and carers towards professionals can manifest itself overtly or covertly. Refusal to attend appointments and non-engagement can appear passive or forgetful, which is concerning in itself, but can also be part of a deliberate strategy to avoid services. Complaints and threats to sue professionals, or even direct threats of violence or assaults on staff, can also subvert the main task of safeguarding children.

Child out of sight and out of mind

Work by Brandon (2009) has highlighted concerns about children somehow falling "out of sight and out of mind". Often this is startlingly literal—professionals have somehow been obstructed from actually seeing or accessing children and fail to attribute the appropriate concern to such deliberate impediments. In other cases the child is "seen" yet somehow "not seen", perhaps because the mother's problems regarding her health or current housing appear repeatedly to dominate the agenda with professionals.

Abuser out of sight and out of mind

Although younger children may somehow be "out of sight and out of mind", in contrast adolescent victims of abuse may be very visible and well known to services for problems such as self-harm or depression; yet they do not disclose the abuse for reasons such as shame or wishing to protect the abuser. In youth offending services or prison settings the focus can be on the young person as a perpetrator of an offence, rather than on their past or ongoing victimisation, potentially driven by ongoing intimidation from others preventing disclosure. There has recently been a general increase in awareness regarding gang-related sexual exploitation of young people of both sexes.

Disgust towards the child

Clinicians and professionals who work with children have usually chosen to work in the field with a sense of vocation and a desire to help children and families. Although there is variation between disciplines, professional training programmes typically encourage the development of warm and empathic client interactions. The clinical reality of service users, who may be challenging, unkempt, and unpleasant, can come as a shock. It can be particularly difficult for individuals who aspire to be caring clinicians to admit to feelings of disgust at a young person due to their physical condition, individual characteristics, or the offences they have committed (e.g., sexual offences).

Professional anxiety and fear of being blamed

Some high-risk cases can generate such elevated levels of fear and anxiety that individuals feel unable to cope. These fears may be less related to actual risks posed by patients or clients and more related to the fear of scrutiny and criticism by supervisors or inspectors if any untoward event were to happen. Such anxieties can lead to the premature discharge of young people from services and a genuine subsequent increase in risk and failure to support that young person. Similarly, the fear of acting with excessive coercion or restriction can cause clinicians to withhold from delivering necessary or effective interventions for young people, including safeguarding interventions.

Such mechanisms, operating at conscious or unconscious levels, can effectively derail the central task of safeguarding children. They can also interfere with the therapeutic delivery of children's services in our partner agencies, especially when individuals and supervisors are structure or task-oriented and not equipped to manage the interpersonal demands of service delivery.

> A female youth offending service case worker described a session with a young person during which the young person made a sexual advance towards her—which she declined, and tried to ignore, but which she found extremely unsettling. On sharing this incident with her supervisor, she was asked, "Why are you telling me this?" In the absence of any other support, she felt unable to work with this young person and questioned whether she should stay in her current job.

Group-related challenges in multiagency work

Following an assessment typically conducted by an individual, the main arena for making decisions on child protection matters in England and Wales is the multiagency meeting, which aims to include a wide range of relevant professionals including mental health professionals.

However, these meetings introduce potential difficulties at a group level that merit some discussion. The "Abilene paradox", as documented by Harvey (1974), describes the bizarre situation in which a group can jointly decide a course of action that on later reflection was actually not actively supported by anyone in the group but was nonetheless agreed via a process that included ambivalent proposals from one member and a degree of deference and uncritical agreement by others. Another proposed challenge is that of "groupthink" (Janis, 1982) in which the strong wish to maintain group cohesion can result in alternative proposals not being explored and novel options not being considered for fear of differences harming or destroying the group.

There is a considerable volume of research literature on group processes and decision-making. In the emotive field of child protection, it is not unusual for heated discussions between professionals to erupt, sometimes due to significantly differing or opposing views regarding risk and management plans.

Towards therapeutic multiagency work

In the effort to improve services for the protection of children from abuse, the outcomes of Serious Case Reviews have been explored in detail (Brandon, Sidebotham, Bailey, & Belderson, 2010) with numerous recommendations for reform and development of children's services (Munro & Hubbard, 2011; Social Care Institute for Excellence, 2010).

Of note, The Munro Review of Child Protection highlights that;

> the emotional dimension of working with children and families plays a significant part in how social workers reason and act. If it is not explicitly discussed and addressed then its impact can be harmful. It can lead to distortions in social workers' reasoning because of the unconscious influence it has on where attention is focused and how information is interpreted. (Munro, 2011, p. 91)

Ferguson (2005) and Ingram (2012) emphasise the need for a "psycho-social perspective" and "emotional intelligence" at the heart of social care to help deliver effective services. They draw attention to the significant emotional challenges and obstacles in routine social work, including very real threats of violence. In this context, it appears that there is a great deal to be gained from the insights provided by psychology and psychotherapy in helping professionals work with the vivid emotional and interpersonal challenges of child protection work. For example, the seemingly "incomprehensible" abuse of children by their parents can be disorientating, and we no doubt benefit enormously from the pioneering work of clinicians such as Winnicott (1949) and Welldon (1988) who help provide a theoretical framework with which to work therapeutically with perpetrators and victims of childhood maltreatment. In many respects, child protection is a thoroughly "forensic" task.

The significant challenge we continue to face is one of service delivery: how to integrate and share this knowledge and expertise to enrich and shape the practice of colleagues in partner agencies. There are several models for delivery of mental health services in collaboration with partner agencies, as described earlier, and the trend towards increasing integration and collaborative cross-agency work will continue to open new possibilities for sharing skills and developing therapeutic approaches.

The Interpersonal Dynamics (ID) consultation and child protection

The ID consultation described by Reiss and Kirtchuk (2009) is a helpful framework that can help deliver these objectives. It offers a structured format for client-centred reflective practice which has been used for many years in forensic psychiatric settings. The strengths of the ID consultation include its accessibility to all disciplines and all levels of seniority, its jargon-free content and its reflective non-blaming approach. It can be incorporated into a team's routine clinical practice and facilitates information gathering that complements and enhances existing risk assessments.

The ID consultation was recently piloted in a multiagency safeguarding setting with the aim of enhancing multiagency working in order to generate a shared formulation and management plan. A particularly helpful aspect has been the way in which staff have been supported to identify and express emotions: given permission "to think and say the unthinkable and unsayable".

Case study

A six-year-old white British girl alleged that her twelve-year-old brother had perpetrated penetrative sexual abuse on her, leading to his arrest. The mother of the children presented as "respectable and middle class"; she calmly but forcefully resisted police enquiries, and the allegations of sexual abuse were soon retracted by the six-year-old girl. The mother of the two children blamed evil spirits for causing the girl to invent such a story, and the police took no further action.

The twelve-year-old boy was clearly extremely anxious and traumatised. Background information regarding sexual abuse of the twelve-year-old boy came to the attention of professionals, together with accounts of the mother's violent and criminal behaviour that appeared to be out of keeping with her hitherto calm presentation—and the apparently unexplained death "due to natural causes" of another young child some years before. The mother explosively denied any difficulties with the current two children.

In a short period of time, a gulf of opinion formed between the child protection social worker, who deemed the mother to be a good parent, and child mental health professionals who raised grave concerns. The safeguarding concerns raised by the mental health team were met

> with ferocity by the mother, who threatened to assault and sue clinicians; and she refused to allow her son to attend further therapeutic sessions. The social worker firmly aligned himself with the mother and accused the mental health worker of being unprofessional and not knowing how to work with children.

An ID consultation was called to help make sense of this gridlock. Relevant individuals with first-hand experience and senior social work managers were invited to discuss the case using the ID cluster list. The comments made during the consultation are summarised in Figure 2 below.

A. The client repeatedly perceives others as:	
The mother was quoted as saying:	
<u>To the child mental health team:</u>	
"You're accusing me" "You're saying I've done something to my children"	*Accusing*
"You are telling me how to live my life"	*Domineering and imposing*
"You are destroying this family" "You are trying to remove my children" "I'm going to sue you"	*Intimidating and attacking*
<u>To the social worker:</u>	
"You agree with me—you don't have any concerns about me"	*Behaving as though she knows best*
B. The client regularly experiences his/herself as:	
The mother was quoted as saying:	
"I know what's best for my kids"	*Behaving as though she knows best*
"I'm refusing to leave the room" "I'm not like that—why do think I'm aggressive?"	*Defying and opposing*
"I'm doing the best I can"	*Attending to and caring*
"You are traumatising me" "You have ruined my life"	*Indignant and self-justifying*

(*Continued*)

C. Others/staff regularly perceive the client as:	
The child mental health team reported:	
"She threatened to sue me and shouted at me"	*Intimidating and attacking*
"The mother lies all the time"	*Manipulating and exploiting*
Social services staff reported:	
"She's a caring mother doing her best"	*Attending to and caring*
"I don't have parenting concerns about her"	*Self-sufficiently independent*
D. Others/staff regularly perceive themselves as:	
The child mental health team reported:	
"Heck, I've got to see her today"	*Giving up in despair*
"The mother is preventing therapy, I have to keep pushing"	*Constantly opposing*
"She is a terrible mother, the worst in the world. I am disgusted by her, it's true"	*Showing disgust*
The social worker's views were:	
"I agree with the mother—therapy doesn't seem to be helpful"	*Supporting and agreeing*
"I let her get on, she's managing things"	*Treating her as self sufficiently independent*

Figure 2. Comments made during the ID consultation.

The first and perhaps the most striking observation at the conclusion of the ID consultation was that the entire discussion had focused on the *mother*. The client was exclusively considered to be the *mother* with no mention at all of the children in any of the four perspectives. The children were well and truly "out of sight and out of mind" at this meeting with no accounts of a child's perspective or staff perspectives towards a child. This excessive focus on the mother meant that the children had disappeared once again.

Second, the significant differences of opinion that were expressed effectively amounted to a polarisation of views; the social worker aligned with the mother whilst the child mental health professional was uncompromisingly concerned about the children's immediate wellbeing. The ID consultation helped identify some of the factors that had led to this, not least the mother's furious attacks on multiple professionals and blocking access to her children. This caused concern in individuals of several agencies and disciplines including teachers, but it appeared that they did not always have a suitable framework for managing or responding to the intense interpersonal challenges. For example, to admit to having difficulty coping with a case may be considered by some to be an admission of weakness and inability to perform one's job, rather than to be a sign of insightful, accurate risk assessment, and maturity.

The information gained from the ID consultation formed the basis of a formulation in which the multiple perspectives contributed to an understandable dysfunctional cycle in the professional network.

The mother experienced the social worker as treating her as though she knows best, which reinforced the mother's perception of herself as indeed knowing best. This was further supported by the social worker's experience of the mother as caring for the children and being self-sufficiently independent, and the social worker's perception of himself as supporting and agreeing with the mother.

In contrast, the mother experienced mental health staff as accusing, domineering, and intimidating, whilst perceiving herself as defying and opposing towards staff and attending to and caring towards her children. This position caused staff to experience the mother as intimidating, attacking, and manipulative, whilst staff perceived themselves as disgusted, wanting to give up in despair, and constantly opposing her. This in turn increased the mother's own experience of defying and opposing staff whom she perceived as domineering.

Finally, the formulation gained from the ID consultation contributed to an enhanced risk formulation and a robust, coordinated multiagency safeguarding plan with a therapeutic mental health component. The ability of this mother to distort the perspectives of professionals and derail safeguarding and therapeutic intervention, including blocking access to the children, was itself a risk that required documentation. The ID consultation also highlighted the mother's own potential adult safeguarding and mental health needs.

Conclusion

Within teams and in a multiagency context, the ID consultation provides a framework for a manageable degree of emotional openness and reflection on the mental states of ourselves and others which helps promote trust and maintain a therapeutic professional relationship with clients. By sharing personal experiences of working with challenging young people and families, professionals feel validated and acknowledged, and the intensity of that emotion can be used to enhance the understanding and needs of the client.

Crucially, the ID consultation can also highlight particular gaps in knowledge, such as when the young person is out of sight and out of mind, or to highlight occasions when the primary task of safeguarding has been subverted. Such findings should be added to risk assessments, since it is precisely in those cases where assessment has been obstructed or subverted and where chaos appears to have taken hold of the network that particularly high risks may lie.

References

Borum, R., Bartel, P. A., & Forth, A. E. (2003). *Manual for the Structured Assessment of Violence Risk in Youth (SAVRY)*. Florida, FL: University of South Florida.

Brandon, M. (2009). Child fatality or serious injury through maltreatment: Making sense of outcomes. *Children and Youth Services Review, 31*: 1107–1112.

Brandon, M., Sidebotham, P., Bailey, S., & Belderson, P. (2010). A study of recommendations arising from serious case reviews 2009–2010. *Research Report DFE-RR157*. UK: Department for Education.

Department for Education. (29 October 2014). *Characteristics of Children in Need in England, 2013–2014*. London: Department for Education. www.gov.uk/government/statistics/characteristics-of-children-in-need-2013-to-2014 [last accessed 15 July 2015].

Department for Education. (26 March 2015). *Working Together to Safeguard Children. A Guide to Inter-agency Working to Safeguard and Promote the Welfare of Children*. London: Department for Education. www.gov.uk/government/publications/working-together-to-safeguard-children--2 [last accessed 15 July 2015].

Department of Health. (2003). *The Victoria Climbié inquiry: Report of the inquiry by Lord Laming*. London: The Stationery Office.

Easton, M. (17 September 2013). *BBC News—Daniel Pelka: The Mistakes we Keep Making*. London: BBC. www.bbc.co.uk/news/uk-24129865 [last accessed 15 July 2015].

Ferguson, H. (2005). Working with violence, the emotions and the psycho-social dynamics of child protection: Reflections on the Victoria Climbie case. *Social Work Education, 24*: 781–796.

Haringey LSCB. (2009). Serious case review: baby Peter. www.haringeylscb.org/sites/haringeylscb/files/executive_summary_peter_final.pdf [last accessed 18 May 2016].

Harvey, J. (1974). Managing agreement in organizations: the Abilene paradox. *Organizational Dynamics, 3*: 63–80.

Gray, D., & Watt, P. (2013). Giving victims a voice. A joint MPS and NSPCC report into allegations of sexual abuse made against Jimmy Savile under Operation Yewtree. www.nspcc.org.uk [last accessed 18 May 2016].

Ingram, R. (2012). Locating emotional intelligence at the heart of social work practice. *British Journal of Social Work, 2012*: 1–18.

Janis, I. L. (1982). *Groupthink: Psychological Studies of Policy Decisions and Fiascoes*. Boston, MA: Houghton Mifflin.

Local Government Information Unit/Children's Services Network. (2013). Police briefing. Daniel Pelka Serious Case Review. Coventry: LSCB. www.lgiu.org.uk [last accessed 18 May 2016].

Ministry of Justice and Youth Justice Board for England and Wales. (29 January 2015). *Youth Justice Annual Statistics for 2013 to 2014 for England and Wales*. London: Ministry of Justice and Youth Justice Board for England and Wales. www.gov.uk/government/statistics/youth-justice-annual-statistics-2013-to-2014 [last accessed 15 July 2015].

Munro, E. (2011). *The Munro Review of Child Protection: Final Report*. London: Department for Education.

Munro, E., & Hubbard, A. (2011). A systems approach to evaluating organisational change in children's social care. *British Journal of Social Work, 41*: 726–743.

Office for National Statistics. (12 February 2015). Violent crime and sexual offences—homicide. In: *Crime Statistics, Focus on Violent Crime and Sexual Offences, 2013/14*. London: Office for National Statistics. www.ons.gov.uk/ons/rel/crime-stats/crime-statistics/focus-on-violent-crime-and-sexual-offences--2013-14/rpt-chapter-2.html [last accessed 15 July 2015].

Reiss, D., & Kirtchuk, G. (2009). Interpersonal dynamics and multidisciplinary teamwork. *Advances in Psychiatric Treatment, 15*: 462–469.

Smith, C., & Thornberry, T. P. (1995). Relationship between childhood maltreatment and adolescent involvement in delinquency. *Criminology, 33*: 451–481.

Social Care Institute for Excellence. (2010). *Piloting the SCIE "Systems" Model for Case Reviews: Learning from the North West of England*. UK: Social Care Institute for Excellence.

United Nations Convention on the Rights of the Child (UNCRC). (1990). www.ohchr.org/EN/ProfessionalInterest/Pages/CRC.aspx [last accessed 18 May 2016].

Webster, C. D. (1997). *HCR-20: Assessing Risk for Violence*. British Columbia: Mental Health, Law and Policy Institute, Simon Fraser University and Forensic Psychiatric Services Commission of British Columbia.

Welldon, E. V. (1988). *Mother, Madonna, Whore: The Idealization and Denigration of Motherhood*. London: Karnac.

Winnicott, D. W. (1949). Hate in the countertransference. *International Journal of Psychoanalysis, 30*: 69–74.

CHAPTER SEVEN

Consulting on Oedipus: then and now

Aikaterini Papaspirou and Jose Maret

Act I: Oedipus past

This is a consultation to the city of Thebes following the unravelling of Oedipus as described in *Oedipus Rex* (a.k.a. *Oedipus the King* or *Oedipus Tyrannus*), a play written by Sophocles around 430–425 BC. The consultation is instigated by the challenge posed for the people of Thebes in terms of managing and processing the impact of Oedipus and his actions on their minds.

We are informed that plague has spread over the city of Thebes. Oedipus, the King of Thebes, has sent Creon, his wife's brother, to the Oracle of Apollo at Delphi for advice on what he would need to do for the plague to stop. He receives the instruction that he should drive the corruption from the land by banishing or killing Laius' murderer—Laius was Oedipus' predecessor who had been killed and whose wife Oedipus has married. Oedipus seeks further advice from Tiresias, a blind Oracle, in order to identify who the killer is. Tiresias initially wishes to refrain from revealing the truth considering its potential impact on Oedipus and on himself; however, when Oedipus persists in a forceful and disrespectful manner Tiresias states that he, Oedipus, had murdered Laius. Oedipus reacts in an angry and dismissive way expressing the belief that Creon has conspired with Tiresias against him. Tiresias goes on to indicate that Laius' murderer is a native Theban, one who has borne children with his own mother. Oedipus confronts Creon convinced he is scheming against him and is responsible for Tiresias' allegation that Oedipus has killed Laius.

Jocasta, Oedipus' wife, intervenes along with the Chorus to bring reconciliation between Creon and Oedipus. She disputes the Oracle's capacity to see into the future and offers as proof that Laius had been told by an Oracle that he would die from the hand of their son but was reported to have been killed by thieves at a place where three roads meet; moreover, Laius had fastened with pins his three-day-old son's ankles and had given him to a henchman to leave on a barren mountain. Oedipus is shaken and asks about the place and the time of Laius' killing as well as for details of what had happened. We discover that Oedipus was raised in the nearby city of Corinth by King Polybus and Queen Merope. When doubt was cast on Oedipus' heritage and despite his parents' angry response to his questioning about this, he sought clarification from the Delphi Oracle only to be told that he was going to kill his father and couple with his mother. He then decided not to return to Corinth to prevent this prophecy from coming true. Furthermore, before arriving at Thebes Oedipus reached a place where three roads meet where he killed a man on a wagon; this man—who matched Laius' description—was escorted by a herald and along with his wagon driver attempted to thrust Oedipus off the road.

As Oedipus begins to consider he might in fact be Laius' murderer, a messenger from Corinth comes to announce that King Polybus is dead. Oedipus remains concerned that even if his father's death did not come as a result of his killing him he might partially fulfil the prophecy by marrying Merope, his mother. The messenger, however, informs him that he was not Polybus' and Merope's biological son but had been given to the King of Corinth by himself who was a shepherd at the time and who had received Oedipus from a shepherd from Laius' court. The story comes together when the Theban shepherd who had handed baby Oedipus to the Corinthian shepherd and had witnessed Laius' killing confirms under duress that Oedipus had been given to him by Laius *and* Jocasta to be left to die. The realisation that Oedipus has killed Laius and is the son of Laius and Jocasta leads Jocasta to kill herself by hanging while Oedipus blinds himself using Jocasta's brooches following on from finding her dead body.

The timing of the consultation is that of the end of the play. At this stage Creon and the people of Thebes are faced with blind Oedipus, an Oedipus who, as now is common knowledge, had enacted wishes and impulses that according to Freud constitute the universal fantasy of the Oedipus Complex: his murderous wishes and impulses towards one parent (his father) and his incestuous ones towards the other (his mother).

Act II: Interpersonal Dynamics (ID) formulation on Oedipus past

Initially Oedipus appears to experience others as **behaving as though he knows best**: he is aware people seek his advice and intervention in order to free the city of Thebes from the plague. He is the King of Thebes: he acknowledges that his people **accept him and admire him**, and **see him as special**—the world knows his fame, as he states. However, his encounter with Tiresias reveals that he can also rather readily experience others as **accusing** and **attacking of him**: he is convinced that Tiresias is falsely alleging he is Laius' murderer and that Creon is conspiring with Tiresias to overthrow and kill him. He also indicates that fate imposed on him a life of grief. In response to the above Oedipus' perception of himself evolves from that of being a King who **cares and attends** to his people's needs, who **behaves as though he knows best** keeping his people's interest in mind, and who **is special** for having been able to solve the Sphinx's riddle and save Thebes; to coming to recognise himself as **attacking** and destructive—for the first time when it occurs to him the man he had killed in the past was likely to be Laius, and, even more overwhelmingly, when it is confirmed that Laius and Jocasta were his biological parents; and, finally, to that of a man **cutting off contact** both from those he harmed and those he loves by blinding himself, and **giving up in despair** in the face of immense grief and sorrow.

Others' experience of Oedipus reflects a similar pattern: the people of Thebes initially appeal to him as they accept **he sees himself as special**—and for good reason—**he cares for them** and **he behaves as though he knows best**. Through Tiresias and Creon, though, an experience of Oedipus as **domineering and imposing**, as well as **accusing** of others emerges. Again he is only acknowledged as **attacking** when it comes to light that he had killed Laius and that Jocasta killed herself when she realised Oedipus was her son. His act of blinding himself is also experienced as an attack upon himself. By that time the people of Thebes expect Oedipus will **cut off contact** by leaving their city. They have been aware of **accepting and admiring** Oedipus and of **considering him special** and **behaving as though he knew best**; however, they were less able to acknowledge they were **pouring out concerns and anxieties** on to him and were **over-relying upon him**. Maybe at times they also felt compelled to **appease him and comply with him**, especially when he presented as more domineering or as convinced there was a conspiracy against him. Tiresias might have experienced himself as **insisting on his position to the extent of having to defy** Oedipus when he was asked to identify Laius' killer. By the end of the play Creon makes an effort to **attend to** blind, collapsed Oedipus and to show some compassion after he consults the gods. However, we do wonder whether there is also a wish to **cut off contact from** Oedipus by removing him to the palace and ensuring he is exiled from Thebes so as to protect the city from his impact.

Overall, in the course of the play we notice a shift in the relationship of Oedipus to himself and to others: initially there is an experience of Oedipus as an ideal, competent, and reliable ruler to whom his people turn for support and advice, but slowly Oedipus' paranoia and capacity for aggression comes to the fore. As his past connects with his present the realisation of his destructiveness affects himself and others and the wish to disconnect so as to stop this painful experience becomes more prominent. What is less evident is that this disconnection might put Oedipus and the city of Thebes at risk of losing sight of Oedipus' acts of violence and incest and of missing an opportunity to mourn the loss and learn from their experience so this pattern would not be repeated.

Chorus: attacks on the eyes, attacks on the capacity to know: When the Oedipus complex is enacted

Our interest in consulting to Thebes was sparked by our contact over the years with multidisciplinary teams on forensic psychiatric wards in the context of ID consultations. There have been instances when the patient's presentation left us with a strong impression that their index offence was an enactment of their murderous and incestuous impulses towards a rather dysfunctional internalised parental couple. In some cases those impulses are expressed in a particularly concrete manner which brings to mind Oedipus' actions, including his attack on the eyes.

We have been particularly interested in how teams can cut off emotional contact with such patients in a way that can lead to an overestimation of the patient's capacity to function adequately and an underestimation of the patient's risk as expressed in the index offence as well as in analogous behaviour during their admission.

Act III: Oedipus present

The ward team responsible for Mr B's care requests an ID consultation as they have noticed that even though he appears to make good progress on their pre-discharge ward they are left feeling somewhat uneasy about supporting his discharge—while they are positive about discharging him in the near future into the community, this feels "premature". The patient's identity and background have been disguised by creating a composite in order to protect the patient's confidentiality while maintaining the essence of the process and the content of the consultation.

The Team let us know that Mr B is a man in his early twenties. He has been diagnosed with schizoaffective disorder. He was initially transferred to the medium secure admissions' ward from prison. He was charged with grievous bodily harm for an assault against his mother with whom he was living at the time.

Following his admission Mr B responded quickly to antipsychotic medication. He appeared remorseful about his index offence, and he was keen to engage in activities and to undergo an assessment by the team psychologist. He was soon deemed safe enough to be transferred to a rehabilitation ward and had recently been accepted on a pre-discharge ward. He was frequently described as a "model patient", who would offer advice and support to fellow patients and would try to be of help to staff. Sometimes staff are concerned that he does "too much", for example, he makes an effort to attend all groups available on the ward and engages intensely in psychological therapies; they think he tends to put pressure on himself. On rarer occasions he has been observed to be "pushing boundaries" on the ward, for example, taking on the role of the advocate in relation to other patients' treatment and management.

In terms of his background history the team noted he was an only child and that his parents separated when he was a young teenager: his father left his mother for another woman. Subsequently his mother became rather depressed and used Mr B as her confidant. He initially maintained some contact with his father; however, he stopped this under pressure from his mother. As an adolescent he appeared to gradually lose interest in his schoolwork and to withdraw from the few friends he had; he began using cannabis and spending more time on computer games. His relationship with his mother also deteriorated further: there were frequent fights between them especially with regard to his school performance and his reluctance to help his mother with household chores. Mr B made a brief attempt to move away from the family home when he started college. However, he dropped out and he returned to live with his mother. In the year preceding the index offence he visited his GP with complaints of low mood and was prescribed an antidepressant. During his admission he disclosed that by then he had begun to harbour the belief that his mother was not his mother and that she had been taken over by "innerbodies": he described those as alien creatures "of a different set of dimensions".

By that time we noted that the team had not so far let us know any details about Mr B's index offence. With some reticence they informed us that his assault on his mother involved causing severe injuries on her genitalia with a blunt instrument. When he was arrested he gave an incoherent account of how he attacked his mother to get rid of the "innerbodies". However, when he was assessed by the forensic medical examiner he was not found to be presenting as acutely psychotic and he was remanded in custody. He came to the attention of the prison mental health inreach team a few days later after he attempted to stab himself in the eye with a sharpened pencil: fortunately he was stopped before he could cause severe damage to both eyes but his eyesight had been affected. We thought it was striking that the above information had not been brought up earlier, and we were curious what might have stopped the team from sharing it with us.

In terms of the ID cluster/item list the team said that Mr B believed that others saw him as **self-sufficient** and **treated him as special**, for example, he said that his mother would often turn to him because he was "mature for his age" and could "fend for himself". He also occasionally talked about his mother **ignoring** his needs in that his mother would not notice if he was struggling at school or that he was using cannabis. However, he had also conveyed feeling **put down and humiliated by others**, for example, when staff told him he intervened in other patients' care or when his mother told him off for not helping her at home. On occasions he had also referred to having felt **rejected** by his father who did not make a more active effort to spend time with him when he was growing up. In response to the above Mr B conveyed an experience of himself as **self-sufficient and independent** and as **treating himself as special**: he expressed the view he was able to set up an activity programme for himself without staff's help and that he was very different from other patients on the ward in his capacity to plan his recovery and to help staff help other patients. He saw himself mainly as someone who **would care for others and attend to their needs**, for example, in relation to his mother, fellow patients, and occasionally staff on the ward. There were also times when he saw himself as **insisting on his position**, for example, when he disagreed with staff or his mother.

The team's main impression of Mr B was that he came across as **self-sufficient and independent**, that is, he was more able to manage his frustrations on his own compared with other patients and that he didn't need that much input. They often found him **defying and opposing** but also occasionally **superficially compliant and appeasing** when it came to negotiating with him care plans and putting to him their concern that he might overwhelm himself by engaging in too many therapeutic activities. It was highlighted that the team found it difficult to consider that Mr B could be **intimidating and attacking** towards others, that is, towards his mother, the victim of his index offence, but also towards himself—it was at this stage that it came to light that there had been instances when Mr B presented as perplexed, distraught, and mumbling to himself: during such periods he made attempts to take his eyes out and received increased support by ward staff but did not have the dose of his antipsychotic medication increased. His care team experienced themselves as **treating Mr B as special**—a "model patient". They felt they **attended to and cared for him in every way** and also at times noticed that they could become **overinvolved**, feeling sorry for him for being in hospital given his young age. They expressed concerns they might be **opposing him** as they were wondering whether they were slowing down his progress towards discharge by not providing more activities for him. However, they found it more difficult to consider they might have also been **appeasing him** at times when they had given in to his requests while they were somewhat worried whether he was taking on more that it would be good for him. When we brought to their attention that it was possible that they **were cutting off contact** from the horror of his index offence and of the damage he had inflicted upon his eyes, as indicated by their reluctance to discuss those aspects of his presentation earlier in the consultation, we were met with bemusement.

Chorus: Steiner's concept of turning a blind eye

John Steiner, psychoanalyst, explores Oedipus Rex in his paper "Turning a blind eye: The cover up for Oedipus" (1985). Steiner considers that Oedipus (but also other participants in the drama) might have been aware of the evidence leading to the truth but had resorted to covering it up—they had *turned a blind eye* to it. He describes that the incestuous and murderous feelings which arise as a result of feeling jealous in relation to the parental couple can be evaded and covered up leading to a partial misrepresentation and distortion of reality. This would protect the individual from having to face the phantasy crimes against the parental couple and process the concomitant feelings of guilt and fear. However, this defensive manoeuvre leaves the individual in fear of the cover-up being exposed and in need to perpetuate it so as to prevent an internal collapse. According to Steiner the mechanisms involved in turning a blind eye include the use of *chance* as a way of denying the conclusion arising from the available evidence—believing there is a chance that the initial observation has not been proven against all doubt and that things might mean something else despite the evidence—as well as *collusion*: believing something against the evidence of one's senses because it is convenient to do so. He is of the view that turning a blind eye stems from an organisation of defences related to a borderline psychotic attitude towards reality and links it to the split described by Freud in his paper on fetishism (1927).

We consider that the concept of turning a blind eye and its link to collusion is relevant to our experience of how the vicious circles of interpersonal dynamics emerging in our consultations are maintained. In fact it appears that when it is no longer possible to continue turning a blind eye cutting off contact becomes the alternative.

ACT IV: the vicious circles of tragedies

As far as Oedipus is concerned we notice that once his more tyrannical and destructive aspects come to the fore the initial pattern of an idealising relationship between him and the people of Thebes collapses. Owning up fully to the knowledge of Oedipus' actualised murderous and incestuous impulses becomes too much for everybody. The task would have been one of managing the overwhelming emotions through a process of collective mourning, of acknowledging the losses and failures and attempting to understand why Oedipus became who he was and why the people of Thebes turned a blind eye to the circumstances surrounding his becoming the King. However, Oedipus and the people of Thebes resort to cutting off contact, disconnecting from Oedipus' actions and of their horrendous emotional consequences. This creates a situation in which neither Oedipus nor the people over whom he ruled learn from their experience or face their limitations in a way that would allow them to develop a more objective appraisal of reality. But this would be subject matter for other Greek tragedies detailing the end of Oedipus' life (*Oedipus at Colonus*) and the fate of the rulership of Thebes (*Seven against Thebes, Antigone*).

In Mr B's case the pattern which is repeated is that of his presenting and being treated as prematurely self-sufficiently independent and as someone who is expected to provide and care for others; this is constantly reinforced to the patient's detriment. His pseudo-mature presentation is closely linked to his reported experience of having been used by his mother as a substitute for his father following his parents' separation. In a sense Mr B became a King in his father's place and was left with his mother as his partner. As much as this fulfilled at some level a fantasy of killing the father and coupling with the mother, it also deprived Mr B of the opportunity to be cared for in an age-appropriate manner and to develop psychosexually in a more ordinary way. Similarly on the ward he becomes more identified with the role of staff members rather than allowing himself to be a patient with a history of a severe mental illness and violence who is in need of care and support in order to recover. The ward team turn a blind eye to Mr B's predicament by accepting his precociousness even though at times they register a feeling of concern for him. However, noticing and thinking about his propensity for violence towards others as well as towards himself is rather challenging.

Our impression was that the ward team found it rather painful to integrate in their minds their experience of an apparently competent but neglected young man with that of a psychotic patient capable of inflicting severe injuries on his mother's body and on his own eyes; they, therefore, cut off contact from the more disturbing aspects of his presentation and history with the result of unwittingly reinforcing Mr B's pseudo-maturity and sense of self-sufficiency and perpetuating the neglect of his mental health needs. We felt that this also affected the team's ability to assess objectively Mr B's risk of harm to others and to himself, making them prone to underestimate its severity and the need for long-term management of such risk.

Exodus: Oedipus and the value of consultation

We often find ourselves wondering why teams of experienced and competent mental health professionals might face difficulties in keeping a balanced view of patients like Mr B—why they might collude with such patients' defensive structures in a way that prevents them from being able to realistically assess the patients' level of functioning, resources, and risks. The following verses from *Oedipus Rex* capture some of our thoughts on this:

> I pity you but I can't bear to look.
> I've much to ask, so much to learn,
> So much fascinates my eyes,
> But you … I shudder at the sight. (Sophocles, tr. R. Fagles, 1984, p. 239)

These are the Chorus' remarks upon seeing Oedipus following his act of self-blinding. Oedipus' appearance at that very moment is the culmination of his transgressions, of his acts of violence and incest. He has turned himself into a horrendous vision. The Chorus is filled with horror at this sight—but also overwhelmed with fascination and curiosity.

Perhaps we are caught up in a similar emotional paradox when we are faced in our clinical practice with patients who have concretely transgressed the Oedipal taboo with their offences, who have enacted the very wishes and impulses we have repressed. As much as we might have been able to negotiate our conflicts in relation to our experience of a parental couple and internalised a more or less benign version of it which would allow us to keep a broader view of ourselves and others, there still remains an area of unresolved murderous and incestuous desires and impulses within us. This renders us vulnerable to becoming both fascinated and horrified by the permutations of the Oedipal tragedies enacted by forensic patients, and it can compel us to turn a blind eye or cut off contact emotionally. Hopefully an ID consultation can provide a safe space in a clinical setting for such emotions to be acknowledged and processed within a care team in a way that would help us to continue engaging genuinely with our patients for their benefit.

References

Fagles, R., Sophocles, & Knox, B. (1984). *The Three Theban Plays: Antigone; Oedipus King; Oedipus at Colonus*. London: Penguin Books, Kindle edition.

Freud, S. (1927). Fetishism. In: J. Stachey (Ed. & Trans.), *The Standard Edition of the Complete Psychological Works of Sigmund Freud* (Vol. 21). London: Hogarth Press.

Steiner, J. (1985). Turning a blind eye: The cover up for Oedipus. The *International Review of Psycho-analysis, 12*: 161–172.

CHAPTER EIGHT

Training ID consultants: a fertile matrix

John Gordon, Richard Ingram, and Gabriel Kirtchuk

Forensic psychotherapy is the application of a psychoanalytic perspective to clinical work with the most severely ill, difficult, and at times frightening patients in secure and community settings. The training matrix within which it developed has deep and wide historical roots. Mervyn Glasser, Adam Limentani, Robert Hale, Donald Campbell, and Estela Welldon at the Portman Clinic, among many others working independently such as Arthur Hyatt-Williams and Patrick Gallwey, have made major contributions. Murray Cox and Leslie Sohn at Broadmoor Hospital, along with their colleagues, expanded understanding of complex forensic psychopathology in the high secure hospital. The International Association of Forensic Psychotherapy, spearheaded by Estela Welldon, enabled larger gatherings of professionals in the field to present their clinical work and extend their skills. The purpose of this chapter is to indicate some other current, significant components of this fertile matrix and to describe aspects of the resulting training structures and opportunities for clinicians working in this complex area. We intend particularly to specify the necessary context within which trainees may begin to generate a capacity to understand thoroughly and to facilitate Interpersonal Dynamics (ID) consultations.

Origins of a national forensic psychotherapy training structure

In 1997 an inquiry into the Personality Disorder Unit at Ashworth Special Hospital was commissioned following allegations by a patient of serious and pervasive boundary violations. These alleged breaches of care and security included "the misuse of drugs and alcohol, financial irregularities, possible paedophile activity and the availability of pornographic material on the Unit" (Department of Health, 1999, Peter Fallon's letter to the Secretary of State). The allegations were found "to be largely accurate. Pornography was widely available on the ward; patients were running their own businesses; Hospital policies were ignored; and security was grossly inadequate" (ibid.). Scathingly, the inquiry concluded that "The PDU was a deeply flawed creation. A number of highly serious reports have demonstrated Ashworth Hospital's failure to care for and manage a large group of severely personality disordered patients" (ibid.). Finally—and crucially for the training developments traced in this account—the committee members emphasised deficits in the capacity to formulate and think about (in effect, to contain) the emotional turbulence of contact with severe personality disorder: "The focus of clinical discussion and decision-making was predominantly on social behaviour and administrative and risk issues, rather than on seeking a psychological understanding of the patient" (Department of Health, 1999, 4.2.27).

In response to this emergency and these clinical concerns, Robert Hale from the Portman Clinic was influential in negotiating with the Department of Health the establishment of nine five-year dual training posts in forensic psychotherapy (psychiatry). Subsequently, West London Mental Health NHS Trust joined the Portman Clinic to add a further two posts.

Doctors with a dual training in forensic psychiatry and psychoanalytic psychotherapy would be much better equipped to enhance multidisciplinary teams' awareness of the often unconscious dynamics arising from patients' early experiences and to consider the reverberating emotional impacts which determined relationships between patients and professionals on the wards and in other mental health settings. Accordingly, the "psychological understanding of the patient" underlined by the committee could be addressed. However, such a small number of isolated psychodynamically informed clinicians spread across the UK required the development of a peer group to consolidate their identity in this new specialty as well as to provide continuing training. Consequently, with the support of the Department of Health (particularly Eddie Kane) and of the Royal College of Psychiatrists, the National Strategy for Forensic Training and Education chaired by Gill McGauley together with Gabriel Kirtchuk as lead clinician was formed to support the dual trainees and to anticipate and meet subsequent training requirements.

In retrospect, the next phase was obvious: the relatively small number of medical trainees would never expand to the point of creating a critical mass of psychodynamically skilled professionals who could have a decisive impact within forensic services. Therefore, a proposal to develop a pilot project for a multidisciplinary training leading to a forensic practitioner level qualification was considered by the National Strategy. The Forensic Psychotherapy Department at West London NHS Mental Health Trust took on this project based on another key aspect of the matrix we are describing: a prolonged experience within the Trust of using basic psychoanalytic concepts to teach a wide range of multidisciplinary professionals. This strand of the matrix, long predating the Ashworth inquiry with which our story began, will now be described.

The MSc

The two-year MSc in Psychotherapeutic Approaches in Mental Health is a collaboration between the Forensic Psychotherapy Training Department at West London Mental Health NHS Trust and New Buckinghamshire University. This training for multidisciplinary professionals working in general and forensic psychiatric hospitals, community mental health, and associated services (social services, general practice, probation) applies a psychoanalytic perspective to understand the individual, group, and organisational dynamics which permeate their work. In particular, the focus is on how to conceptualise, bear, and use the ubiquitous emotional impacts which unconsciously affect interpersonal relationships at all levels of the clinical setting.

The current MSc is the culmination of a long development which originated in Bob Hinshelwood's Psychotherapy Department at St Bernard's Hospital. In the late 1980s, Bob, David Riley, and John Gordon organised training at the request of the on-site School of Nursing which offered nurses an opportunity to experience and learn about group dynamics and group psychotherapy. Students attended an experiential group, reading seminars, and a residential group relations event modelled on the Leicester conference. Subsequently Gabriel Kirtchuk joined the Psychotherapy Department and devised a Training in Psychodynamic Assessment to which Bob Hinshelwood, David Riley, and John Gordon also contributed. In 1996 Bob left St Bernard's to take up the position of Medical Director of the Cassel Hospital, but a major elaboration of these early ventures then took shape led by Gabriel Kirtchuk, now Consultant Psychotherapist and Head of the Forensic Psychotherapy Department. Nurses had become much more interested in trainings with an academic qualification, so Gabriel, along with John Gordon and Beatrice Stevens, began negotiations with Ellen Noonan, Head of the Counselling Section at Birkbeck College, University of London. After about a year they established a Certificate/Diploma in Work with the Mentally Ill in Hospital and Community, subsequently and even more awkwardly renamed the Certificate/Diploma in Individual, Group, and Organisational Dynamics in Work with the Mentally Ill in Hospital and Community. Although not involved directly in the planning, Bob Hinshelwood (soon to be the first external examiner for the West London/Birkbeck Certificate/Diploma) remained in touch with us throughout. In a letter to Gabriel in June, 1996, he conveyed congratulations and his always thought-provoking reflections on the new venture:

> I want to raise one rather basic issue, which might affect the kind of teaching on the course, and the kind of students who come on it.
>
> As a course primarily for nurses, it seems to me that there might be some space on the course for an "integrative" kind of activity to consider the nurses' medical model approach in relation to the "talking cure" type of approach which the course represents. Working with mentally ill patients is quite a serious and arduous project, and the limits of counselling are obvious. It seems to me that the danger is that nurses can use their new understanding to become, as it were, roving interpreters. As we know, the verbal containing has to take place in a very specific setting. To some extent the question of using psycho-analytically-based insights outside the analytic consulting-room is a research activity … . It seems to me the course might reflect the fundamental difference of approach … and give space for students (and staff) to consider the problems, conflicts and paradoxes that arise. (Hinshelwood, letter to Kirtchuk, June 1996)

We wrestled with this and many other dilemmas involved in teaching applied psychodynamics over the next thirteen years, during which time we were joined by Maya Jarrett from Birkbeck and subsequently by the late Carola Gross from Bob's former psychotherapy department who took over teaching basic psychoanalytic concepts when Beatrice Stevens retired. The course structure remained constant: an academic seminar in which papers from the core psychoanalytic, group and systems theory literature were presented and discussed; an application group in which students presented process accounts of clinical material from work with individual patients and observations of/work in groups, to which the academic concepts and models would be applied; an experiential group; and a group relations event held at Birkbeck College.

At the end of his term, Bob Hinshelwood was succeeded as External Examiner by Marco Chiesa and then Kingsley Norton. Gill McGauley had been the current External Examiner until her recent death. Over 150 students, mainly nurses but also occupational therapists, social workers, "creative" (arts, music, and drama) therapists and a few doctors completed this Certificate/Diploma. Their feedback was always illuminating as the following examples reveal.

A Community Psychiatric Nurse (CPN) in the Elderly Mentally Ill team wrote: "It gave me a lot of insight into working with the anxieties about growing old experienced by my patients and helped me to contain them."

A Care Manager at a Community Mental Health Centre emphasised another aspect:

> The course helped me to understand the group dynamics taking place in my resource centre and to reflect more on the personal impact of the work on myself. It's given me an insight into previously confusing emotional interactions with patients. It's really got me thinking. (Personal communication)

A GP commented:

> I have learned a more meaningful appreciation of human relationships after attending this course and have developed a more searching attitude while solving problems that exist in my clinical practice. The course has given me the confidence to enter into my

> patients' inner worlds to identify emotional reasons for presenting complaints and symptoms. (ibid)

Finally, a Senior Nurse at a Community Mental Health Resource Centre observed:

> Initially it was daunting and I felt, "What is this about?", but as the course went on I began to understand the relevance not only to my work but to my life. Professionally, it's helped to understand personality disordered patients and especially how I am affected by them. (ibid)

Towards the end of what came to be called the "Birkbeck Course" period, once again developments in nursing education prompted a major change in our thinking about the course. Over half of applicants now already had BSc degrees. Accordingly, Gabriel Kirtchuk and John Gordon, joint course organisers, decided to approach Birkbeck College to discuss the scope for expanding the training to BSc or MSc level. After brief talks it became clear that this would not be possible at Birkbeck, so we very regretfully said goodbye to our collaborators of many years. Nursing training had itself moved off-site and was based at Buckinghamshire New University which, because of its educational contract with the Trust, presented itself as a potential new partner. Negotiations with several members of the University administration eventuated in the establishment of the current MSc, and the first student cohort started in September 2010. Core teaching staff included John Gordon, Gabriel Kirtchuk, Maggie McAlister, Ronald Doctor, and Beate Schumacher. A "satellite" development of the MSc in Northern Ireland, led by Richard Ingram with Chris Fry, will be described below.

The curriculum

The current MSc is a two-year course composed of four modules: Psychotherapeutic Approaches to Working with Individuals; Psychotherapeutic Approaches to Working with Groups and Organisations; Interpersonal Dynamics Consultation and Dissertation. The first three modules explicitly envisage the application of psychoanalytic thinking (including attachment and mentalization-based theories) to three key areas with which students, as professional clinicians, are concerned: work with individuals and sometimes with patient groups but always within a group and an institutional dynamic context which both fundamentally shape all interventions within the system.

Module three, the Interpersonal Dynamics (ID) consultation, teaches students a manualised (Kirtchuk, Gordon, McAlister, & Reiss, 2013) protocol for carrying out consultations to ward and community teams. As we have described in previous chapters, individual patients referred for this consultation will usually be causing problems for the multidisciplinary professionals involved in their containment, treatment, and care. The aim of the consultation is to elicit from staff most involved with the patient the core interpersonal patterns regularly evoked in interactions between the patient and her significant others, including the staff, in the present and the past. This is accomplished through applying a structured list of descriptions of how (1) the patient repeatedly perceives others; (2) how the patient in response repeatedly experiences himself; (3) how others repeatedly perceive the patient; and (4) how others in response characteristically experience themselves. These four perspectives basically describe any interpersonal interaction, and the descriptors used are jargon-free. However, it is clear that from the psychodynamic orientation of the MSc we are aiming to provide students with a method of discovering the transference–countertransference scenarios which are unconsciously enacted and re-enacted by the patient and others. These scenarios are often profoundly maladaptive, however entrenched their defensive functions, and they can evoke equally maladaptive, even destructive, automatic reactions from staff. Alerting staff to their potential for such reactions by tracing how their patients' impacts are affecting them is a fundamental part of applied psychodynamics. Students are expected to carry out two consultations and to develop increasingly complex formulations of the material to feed back to their teams.

The fourth, Dissertation, module surveys quantitative and qualitative research methods and attempts to introduce psychodynamic aspects of qualitative research such as that exemplified in the work of Wendy Hollway (2001). Qualitative approaches have so far been the predominant choice of students who tend to focus their research on phenomenological accounts of aspects of their work by means of focus groups and semi-structured interviews with mental health staff in their hospital or community settings. This type of research project usually requires only Audit Committee approval and so avoids long delays associated with the Ethics Committee process. Unfortunately, this means that patient-based research is not possible within the short time span of the training, but there have been very interesting studies of, for example, ward reflective practice groups, clinical supervision, and CPN involvement with patients' benefit claims.

The course day

As mentioned above, each teaching day of the MSc is divided into three elements. First students attend an academic seminar in which assigned papers are discussed with a member of the teaching staff. In module one, Psychotherapeutic Approaches to Working with Individuals, these papers from the psychoanalytic literature cover early emotional development and the unconscious mind structured by deficit/conflict, internal working models and internalised self-affect-object relationships, the paranoid-schizoid and depressive positions, splitting and projective identification, transference and countertransference, and the team as container. In module two, Psychotherapeutic Approaches to Working with Groups and Organisations, papers from the wider literature on group dynamics as well as on group therapy are covered. There is a particular focus on projective processes in groups, a theme which is extended when the Tavistock/Group Relations systemic framework for understanding organisations is introduced. Bion's (1961) *Experiences In Groups* is read closely. In module three, papers from the literature on the origins of the ID consultation, internalised self-object relations in personality disorders, perversions and other pathologies, and psychodynamic formulation are discussed. The format is for a student to present a summary of each paper which acts as the launching pad for discussion. Modules three and four run concurrently throughout the second year, and there are academic seminars on research methodology which may also be further discussed in the Application Groups.

The second element of the day is the Application Group. This is a form of work study group made up of five to eight students who in turn present an interaction/session with an individual patient (module one), an observation of a group interaction (module two) or the results of an ID consultation (module three). Every student will have an opportunity to present at least twice during each fifteen-week module. The task of the group is to discuss the presented process account by applying the theories and concepts from the academic seminars to the clinical material. Gradually students become more able to make use of the psychodynamic perspective and to integrate it with the types of treatment interventions inherent in their specific professional roles.

The final element of the day is the Experiential Group. The task of the group is for students to learn about their responses to being a member of a group—how group membership affects the ways in which individuals feel, think, and behave—by getting in touch with and sharing their experiences of the group in the here and now. Wider concerns as members of the course also inevitably emerge in the group meetings.

This combination of academic, clinical, and experiential learning is fundamental to the MSc and links it securely to students' professional roles and responsibilities. Consequently, the MSc is viewed as extremely valuable by trust managers who know from experience how graduates contribute to their ward and community settings as well as to the work of their colleagues.

The MSc lifts off to Northern Ireland

The MSc in Psychotherapeutic Approaches "satellite" training in Northern Ireland has been established now for four years and represents a feasible and effective example of how to develop the opportunity for a multi-professional forensic psychotherapy training in a periphery of the United Kingdom in which there is a relatively modest provision of psychoanalytically trained clinicians.

Approximately seven years ago Richard Ingram, along with interested psychiatry trainees, began travelling on a monthly basis from Belfast to Gabriel Kirtchuk's Forensic Psychotherapy Training Department at West London Mental Health NHS Trust to train in the ID consultation method which had been established there. This association developed further into a weekly teleconferenced workshop in which consultations conducted in London, Belfast, and other interested services in the United Kingdom were discussed and formatted in accordance with the ID consultation model.

Through this contact, psychiatry trainees and other multi-professional staff in Northern Ireland expressed a keen interest in enrolling in the MSc held in London. Funding was found for three candidates who flew over on a rather arduous weekly basis to attend the first year of the course in London. However, through the skills acquired by psychoanalytically trained staff in Belfast in the ID consultation at the weekly workshop, it was decided to run the second year of the course for the Belfast MSc candidates in their home city.

With a small core team of four staff at the Department of Psychotherapy in the Belfast Health and Social Care Trust (Derya Courtney, Chris Fry, Richard Ingram, and Deirdre Meehan), the "satellite" MSc was then established with the help of West London Mental Health NHS Trust and Buckinghamshire New University and now runs with a new intake every two years of ten candidates. Core funding for places was obtained from both the Northern Ireland Department of Health and the local Health and Social Care Board to facilitate applications from multi-professional disciplines working throughout mental health services in Northern Ireland. The funding, which was key to developing and sustaining the training, was obtained in the teeth of the some of the worst funding conditions in the NHS. This was largely as a result of how persuasive the model of training was in terms of developing the innate skills and psychological intelligence available in multidisciplinary teams to maximise the effectiveness of teamwork in managing severely disturbed patients. It was therefore regarded as an investment in education and training which would be significantly cost effective in the medium to long-term.

It is to be hoped that other regions of the United Kingdom may follow in the manner of this successful collaboration, one in which both centres and peripheries can engage in a mutually rewarding experience of high quality service development. The publication of the Interpersonal Dynamics Manual (Kirtchuk, Gordon, McAlister, & Reiss, 2013) and the accessibility of the weekly workshop will now clearly enhance and facilitate potential engagement in this process for other interested regional services. In addition, as will be described shortly, the MSc is now also the initial stage in an escalator model of training for MSc graduates who wish to work towards accreditation as a forensic psychotherapist. This higher level of clinical training is also being designed to be accessible to regions and will therefore also be developed in Northern Ireland as a key element in a strategy to develop and more securely establish forensic psychotherapy as a discipline in this part of the United Kingdom.

Links to the Institute of Group Analysis (IGA), the British Psychoanalytic Council (BPC), and post-MSc qualification

From the inception it was envisaged that the MSc would develop links to psychotherapy training organisations beyond West London Mental

Health NHS Trust and Buckinghamshire New University. Negotiations with the IGA successfully established the first year of the training, based on the module two focus on group dynamics and particularly on the experiential group, as an Introductory (now Foundation) Course equivalent. This enables MSc students who successfully pass year one to apply for full training at the IGA. Inspired by Richard Ingram, further links were made with the BPC which registers graduates of the MSc (who commit themselves to CPD requirements) as psychodynamic practitioners/forensic or general.

A more ambitious proposal builds on all these previous steps and is based on the MSc (or equivalent) as a prerequisite for further training as a multidisciplinary forensic and/or generic psychotherapist as an additional and integrated part of trainees' core clinical profession. The purpose of this training is to increase the number of psychodynamically qualified professionals beyond the current number in order to have a greater impact on increasing demands for talking therapies. Accordingly, we proposed a multi-professional career structure compatible with CPD requirements which encompasses an escalator model of training with valid and registrable stages of experience. There are two stages.

Stage one is the MSc in Psychotherapeutic Approaches in Mental Health (or equivalent) which leads to a qualification as a psychodynamic practitioner/forensic or general approved by the BPC. Following the MSc these trainees will continue within their normal work setting to practice under supervision. In order to increase the psychodynamic orientation of their work, they would be expected to take on specific roles, for example, as co-facilitators of the ward-based Community Meeting, Reflective Practice and ID consultations and to act as supervisors to more junior staff, helping them to understand the dynamics of engagement, relational security, and boundaries from a dynamic point of view. Stage two is a Post-MSc training leading to a qualification as a forensic psychodynamic therapist.

The Forensic Psychotherapy Society

The result of these recent efforts is the birth of a new Member Institution of the BPC, the Forensic Psychotherapy Society, which provides a framework for a national training and multidisciplinary professional pathway in psychodynamic forensic psychotherapy. The aim is to realise the objective, stated above, of establishing a critical mass of skilled professionals who can contribute to a cultural change in our forensic institutions.

References

Bion, W. R. (1961). *Experiences in Groups*. London: Tavistock Publications.

Department of Health. (1999). *Report of the Committee of Inquiry into the Personality Disorder Unit, Ashworth Special Hospital*. London: Department of Health. www.gov.uk/government/uploads/system/uploads/attachment_data/file/265696/4194.pdf [Last accessed 15 September 2015].

Hollway, W. (2001). The psycho-social subject in "evidence-based" practice. *Journal of Social Work Practice, 15*: 9–22.

Kirtchuk, G., Gordon, J., McAlister, M., & Reiss, D. (2013). *Interpersonal Dynamics Consultation: A Manual for Clinicians*. London: www.lulu.com Press.

CONCLUSION

Patient-centred reflective practice

John Gordon and Gabriel Kirtchuk

In the Introduction we presented the Interpersonal Dynamics (ID) consultation within the broader context of reflective practice for staff. As the example there shows, reflective practice groups, like most groups, are often characterised by ubiquitous persecutory anxieties which can so affect relationships among group members as to compromise a focus on effective work or even sabotage the task completely. Further, to stand any chance of becoming a meaningful intervention for mental health and other staff teams, reflective practice must be mandated by senior management. Such authorisation, which means that reflective practice is not voluntary, inevitably enhances group members' suspicion if not conviction (conscious or unconscious) that the facilitator is a management plant or spy who has been sent to gather information which may likely prove extremely detrimental to their careers. That this "paranoid" situation may also be a (projected) reiteration, particularly in forensic, prison, and probation settings, of the patients'/prisoners' core dilemma in confronting their guilt makes it potentially a very useful dynamic to explore in the reflective practice group; but needless to say it also escalates anxiety to the point at which any work at all may cease until these anxieties about the facilitator are faced openly, explored, and at least tentatively resolved. Under the best circumstances this takes considerable determination, resilience, and courage on the part of both staff and facilitators. When in a time of inevitable financial constraint the only stable feature of working life in an organisation is change—change at the levels of service configuration, senior management, and staff ("cuts")—survival anxiety can make the fundamental task of reflecting together on the work even more elusive. In the following concluding pages, we would like to summarise our view of reflective practice in general and to propose the ID consultation as a supplementary form of reflective practice which can help participants to manage their anxieties without distorting the direction of their clinical work.

The basics: "ordinary" reflective practice

Reflective practice is widely accepted as an essential component of good clinical work and has also been called work discussion and staff group supervision. Usually a group of multidisciplinary staff meets regularly (in our service on a weekly basis but in others less frequently) with a facilitator; in other cases the meeting is with a particular professional group. We have had experience of being both external and internal reflective practice facilitators. While external facilitators are inevitably less immersed and so less contaminated by the internal dynamics of the team/organisation with which they meet, it can also be the case that their work becomes encapsulated and split-off from the ongoing work of the clinical team as soon as they leave the room. Internal facilitators face a higher risk of becoming the focus of the persecutory anxieties mentioned above and are as embedded in the life of the setting as other staff (including shared tendencies to collude, evade or take things for granted). But they are also potentially more in touch with the specific and often idiosyncratic internal issues of the organisation and so more aware of the subtle meanings of staff members' communications, especially if they are trained to make use of their countertransference responses. For this reason members of a psychotherapy department or other professionals trained in psychodynamic, group, and systemic processes are likely to be best placed to carry out this role.

Psychopathology and reflective practice

The value, even the indispensability, of reflective practice emerges from an understanding of a frequently encountered form of psychopathology and its effects on patient–staff interactions within mental health settings.

One way to think about our patients is that to a greater or lesser extent they find it hard to manage their own emotional states and those of others around them. At times of strong emotion, they may feel that their perception of a difficult interaction is the only way to see the situation, which may lead to confrontation and dead lock. Or they may characteristically be convinced that their way of seeing things is the only way. This can lead to unbearable tensions in their own minds which are often discharged either through acting out behaviours and boundary breaking or painful and frightening interactions with staff members and other patients which can be hard to reflect upon and address. With forensic patients this is often particularly the case both in their personal histories of previous relationships and in their index offences, which can be thought of as tsunami-like pressures to get rid of unbearable states of mind through action.

This chronic deficit in patients' reflective capacity is naturally expressed in the treatment setting as in all other areas of the patients' lives, past and present. They frequently can't or don't want to know what is going on in their own minds and in their lives, which have frequently been traumatic for themselves and for others. So instead they can behave and talk in certain ways which manage to stir up in other people something like the feelings and thoughts and experiences that they are rarely able to grasp or actively seek to avoid (using the "action mode"). Sometimes just reading a case history might be enough to have a devastating effect on professionals involved in providing care. And this doesn't begin to take account of patients' behaviour on the ward which can at times feel undermining, intrusive or threatening. Consequently, communicating and relating under the conditions of reflective deficit and the action mode are often through emotional (and sometimes physical) impacts on individual members of staff and on the staff team as a whole.

In the treatment setting, patients' difficulties in self-reflection can affect staff in multiple and complex ways. Carrying out a professional role vitally depends on staff finding creative methods to bring together care, treatment, and security in *response—not reaction*—to engagement with patients. The problem is that when patients make emotional impacts on staff the ordinary result can be a human reaction, usually an emotional reaction which may not lead to an action but will certainly be felt strongly by the staff. Many of these emotional impacts are painful, difficult or bewildering. However, whatever goes on in a staff member's mind while relating to a patient might represent a most valuable understanding of what is going on in the patient's mind, especially if it is a patient who doesn't want to or can't understand himself. Some patients may communicate and relate similarly with all members of the Multidisciplinary Team (MDT), while others may have very contradictory effects on different staff. It is only by combining these varied impressions that an in-depth, realistic view of the patient may be reached. Consequently, as individuals and as members of MDTs, professionals need a regular opportunity to stand back and think about the turbulent interactions and impacts which make up everyday life on the wards.

The unique purpose of a Reflective Practice Group is to offer this regular opportunity for staff members to reflect together on their work as individuals and as a team. In particular, by sharing openly their experiences of working with patients and with one another—both positive and negative—professionals may be able slowly to restore the meanings lost to patients. By reflecting on their own responses, staff will be in a better position as individuals to avoid unhelpful and repetitive patterns of interaction and as a team make their multiple interventions more coherent and comprehensible to patients.

Institutional dynamics and reflective practice

Institutions must solve fundamental issues in order to survive and to develop creatively. Primarily, such issues relate to two areas, the primary task and internal organisation. The primary task of an institution is the work it must carry out to justify its existence, the purpose(s) for which it was established in the first place. Depending on the nature of its primary task(s), managers and other members of the institution must work out an internal organisation which facilitates accomplishment of those tasks. Internal organisation of departments, roles, activities, and technical procedures is often referred to by the expression "the division of labour". It would be possible to envisage different divisions of labour for any given primary task, but whatever the internal organisation it must lead to the effective realisation of the primary task(s) and their harmonisation, or at least their mutual non-interference, or the institution will fail.

Primary tasks can be complimentary and also conflictual. For example, a healthcare institution has primary tasks of care, treatment, and security of its patients, as well as training and protection of its staff, but simultaneously it is functioning on behalf of families and society to remove and restrain individuals experiencing feelings or behaving in a manner found to be intolerable or dangerous. In effect, the institution has multiple "clients" and the task of care may compliment/ conflict with the tasks of removal and control. This dilemma could be considered "chronic" when incipient or manifest violence becomes an intrinsic fact of life on the wards because of the nature of the patients' difficulties. Furthermore, treatment and training tasks, complimentary on one level, become conflictual when training requires professionals to move on at a time when treatment considerations mandate continuation of a crucial relationship with the patient: training objectives and patient welfare clash.

Such complementarities/conflicts among primary tasks are the stuff of institutional life, but staff need the opportunity regularly to consider the implications of their actions and decisions in respect to each primary task and to their interactions as well as to work out appropriate internal organisation.

Two examples

Who does what for whom?

On a rehabilitation ward for forensic patients, there is a weekly community meeting at which any issues relating to life on the ward can be raised by patients and staff. A chronic "problem" is the piles of unwashed dishes in the kitchen sink. From the perspective of staff, this constitutes a health risk, a neglect of the primary task of care. It is also a treatment issue; people on a rehab ward, it is said, should be taught to carry out proper hygiene in the kitchen in order to prepare themselves for release to a hostel or other communal living setting. Patients claim that the ward manager is "too soft" on this issue; offending patients—and also sometimes staff—were just plain lazy. A member of staff mentions that when he attempted to call a patient's attention to unwashed dishes, the patient, barely looking him in the face, claimed that he would take no orders from a black man. Another staff member followed up this theme, telling the group that when he asked someone to clean up, he was told by the patient that, "God does not need to listen to people like you." Proposals to lock the kitchen or to deprive miscreants of self catering privileges are made. When explored, it emerges that while such proposals might be in the service of meeting primary tasks of care or even treatment, from another perspective it could also be seen to interfere with the rehabilitative aims of the ward. It was also very unclear why people were not washing up after themselves. Was it laziness; the effects of medication (a view extolled by patients, but viewed by staff as rationalisation); perhaps an indirect expression of protest, aggression, and anger over confinement; a search/demand for a mother figure ("Let the domestic do it, it only takes twenty minutes"); overt racist devaluation; paranoid delusion; or, as the psychotherapist ventures, an expression of the wish not to be "rehabilitated" and so moved on from an environment in which patients had adapted, to a new one which faced them with intolerable anxieties. Did any one of these possibilities underlie the "behaviour", of clear social import to the ward, or was it some combination or an altogether different reason?

What this common example shows is that no immediate "division of labour" to achieve the primary task of rehabilitation—who in which role confronts the patient, what should be said, what options can be presented to the patients—can be determined in advance without systematic reflection on the part of the whole staff team to reach a complex understanding of the reasons for the behaviour and to prioritise their primary tasks on the basis of such understanding.

This complicated work goes beyond the already complex matter of clarifying primary tasks and their interactions, establishing an internal organisation of roles which specify particular activities and interventions, and monitoring whether the "division of labour" is contributing to task performance. The specific work with forensic patients, who are affected by severe mental illness or personality disorder, elicits intense anxieties over personal safety in members of staff. This concern clearly does not only arise in situations of crisis when "untoward incidents" occur. Being in touch daily with disturbed people who have been violent and continue to behave negatively to themselves or others, is itself disturbing and confusing; and everyone has personal means of coping with and defending oneself from emotional disturbance. In addition to individual defensive/coping manoeuvres, groups develop, often unconsciously, ways of operating which serve to protect members from distressing experiences. Such protection is essential, but some forms of protection can be anti-task(s): ways of working are elaborated—out of awareness—which defeat the primary task(s). The reflective practice group must, therefore, also consider such group level hindrances to effective task achievement and help members of staff to devise more adaptively mature personal and communal defences against the anxieties stirred up by the very nature of the work. Otherwise, staff morale as well as task performance suffer and the staff group fragments.

A punch

To illustrate the process of working with communication by impact, consider a reflective practice group for the MDT on a secure forensic ward. Usually attended by a consultant forensic psychiatrist and members of the nursing staff, on this occasion seven nurses, including the ward manager were present. The consultant had not sent apologies, but the group facilitator recalled from another meeting that he had agreed to cover for a colleague who also worked on the ward and was on leave for two weeks. The consultant had expressed considerable apprehension over having to be responsible for all the patients on the ward during this period.

Talk in the group was desultory, and the atmosphere appeared simultaneously tense and fatigued. Eventually the facilitator got the impression that things had been very difficult on the ward with two patients on observation. One of these patients had been particularly threatening. But it was impossible, beyond a general sense of unease and disruption, to get any clear description of what had been happening, how the work had been for individual nurses or what they were feeling about the work.

The facilitator tried several times to indicate his awareness of how hard it had been while also commenting on the prevailing silence in the group. There was little response to his comments until, eventually, a nurse who had presented himself from the start of the reflective practice group as a spokesman for the nurses sharply said, "Why should we talk to someone who only comes for twenty minutes a week? Spend two or three hours on the ward and you'll understand what it's been like!"

This statement felt like a punch to the facilitator, who realised that now he might know something of what the nurses had been feeling over the week. Since his forty-five minute presence for reflective practice had been minimised by over half, it seemed that he represented for the team the absent consultants (both the one on holiday and the one who regularly attended the group). This loss had not been registered—loss rarely is explicitly attended to and thought about in forensic settings—but the facilitator had experienced it in the shape of his ongoing feeling in the reflective practice session that something fundamental was missing in the nurses' own presence and communications.

Paradoxically, the facilitator could simultaneously identify both with the absent consultants and with the staff who were missing them. The "punch" represented the feared reaction of patients to this loss, which staff had been anxiously coping with, now conveyed directly through impact to the facilitator. A further aspect of this situation was that reflective practice—supervision in group form—mobilises what we all feel to some extent when "super"-vised: that a superior figure is looking down on us, probably at the behest of management, to monitor and criticise our work. This is why it is so vital for senior staff to offer examples to their teams of presenting honestly and openly their struggles with the work. It also shows why the reflective practice facilitator must be trained to take and to understand the "punches" of his colleagues.

In the event, the facilitator was able to say that he appreciated the direct comment of the nurse; that he understood that its aggressive punch was related to a picture of him as uninterested and probably critical, but that it also conveyed the depletion of important staff during the week and feelings of anger about additional difficulties which had to be endured over this period. The ward manager and several other members of the group became very active in reassuring the facilitator that the remark had not been meant to be aggressive, that they really appreciated and valued the reflective practice. The facilitator commented that ultimately only frank communication was the best way to value the reflective practice.

Our review and examples demonstrate that for an institution dealing with psychosis and enacted violence, reflective practice is not a slogan but a fundamental necessity for all staff. However, as a means of meeting basic professional and organisational needs, we have also shown how reflective practice groups are intrinsically fraught with complexity and anxiety. Our experience—illustrated in the many examples given in this book—confirms that integrating the ID consultation with "ordinary" reflective practice helps to provide a structured focus, contain the anxiety, and enhance the reflective capacity of both participants and facilitators.

Patient-centred reflective practice

The ID consultation makes a major contribution to development and use of reflective capacity as an essential aspect of clinical practice. From a diagnostic to a treatment planning to a risk management perspective—and particularly in elucidating the most damaged and damaging aspects of the patient—the ID consultation reveals the extent to which clinicians may ignore what is in front of their eyes. For example, item thirteen on the ID cluster list, Intimidating and Attacking (Destroying), is frequently omitted by staff although ample information has been given to make its selection blatantly obvious to the consultant. This omission can have major consequences for the entire strategic overview of a case. For example, premature plans for discharge may be arranged when a patient's delusions regarding his ability to function meet with staff needs to believe they have done a good job, let alone when there are enormous pressures to "unblock" beds. Someone who commits murder and blinds the victim may go on to blind both himself and the staff about his underlying violence, presenting instead a reasonable and compliant attitude. Another patient, seeing himself as highly competent and only needing to take a few computer courses, encouraged staff to believe they had succeeded. As soon as the ID consultation had enabled them to realise the extent of this patient's grandiosity (self-idealisation), staff were able to stand back, reconsider their treatment plan—and the patient immediately became frankly delusional. The ID consultation protects both patient and staff from underestimating the extent of the patient's illness and vulnerability.

The close focus on individual patients and their interpersonal networks both outside and within the treatment setting, inherent in the ID format, helps clinicians formulate a care plan which takes into account the underlying issues of a patient's presentation by offering a more complex understanding of the patient's' and professionals' behaviour, thoughts, and emotions. It also provides a structured task which is more recognisable and therefore congenial in relation to other clinical meetings and practice. This helps to bind group members' anxieties. In addition, the validation given to the views of all members of the multidisciplinary team, including secretaries and domestics—everyone has an experience of relating to the patient which can be a source of valuable information—creates a sense of ownership of the process and the results of the consultation. Not only does such validation bring the team together, but it increases the coherence of treatment plans and interventions which otherwise may become fragmented under the impact of the dysfunctional cycles revealed by the ID consultation.

In regard to the institutional dynamics, a grave problem is lack of integration of treatment (caring) and custodial (coercive) elements inherent in many mental health and prison settings. Both are crucial parts of the primary task; yet they often come to be represented—personified—by different members of the team. When all professionals, including those in managerial and security roles, participate in an ID consultation, it is far more likely that the understandable wish of staff to identify with more humanitarian intentions towards patients, and to disidentify from the coercive qualities of the setting which can be attributed to "management", will not occur. Particularly when staff attempt to elicit patients' perceptions of others (Perspective A), negative reactions to the setting are very likely to emerge. In turn, this enables staff to take greater account of and to own all aspects of the treatment milieu as they are revealed in their estimates of the experiences of their patients. In essence, the ID consultation is a training in "mentalizing" (Bateman & Fonagy, 2004), in formulating a theory of mind: an increasing identification, elaboration, and exploration of the feelings, perceptions, thoughts, and intentions of others, as well as of ourselves. And this is what patient-centred reflective practice should be about.

Reference

Bateman, A. W., & Fonagy, P. (2004). *Psychotherapy for Borderline Personality Disorder: Mentalization-Based Treatment*. Oxford: Oxford University Press.

AFTERWORD

by Colin R. Martin

It is an honour and a pleasure to be asked to write an Afterword for John Gordon's and Gabriel Kirtchuk's excellent book, *Consulting to Chaos*. Reflecting on the wealth of material contained within this comprehensive tome, one is struck by the interplay between theoretical underpinnings, application to practice, and the inclusivity that such an approach to clinical understanding and intervention can potentially offer.

Psychotherapeutic practice, specifically psychodynamic psychotherapy, has, despite an incredibly long, broad, and rich historical backdrop, continued to be viewed by many academics and professionals as a fairly enigmatic approach to both contextualising and intervening with significant mental health disorder. Why might this be the case? Certainly since the revolutionary work of Melanie Klein more than half a century ago, the potential to apply a psychodynamic model to the understanding of, and indeed intervention for, the psychoses has been a core component of the larger psychodynamic armamentarium.

Plausible explanation for this state of affairs in the contemporary context represents a gestalt of service delivery, training, and motivational issues. However, undoubtedly added into this mix must be the availability of a coherent and evidence-based framework that is both accessible to practitioners from a wide range of mental health-related disciplines and offers a process of engaging with patients who experience an extensive range of more severe clinical presentations such as schizophrenia and complex personality disorders, particularly within challenging treatment environments such as forensic psychiatry.

Addressing these issues in a "one-stop" shop volume, John Gordon and Gabriel Kirtchuk have, uniquely, furnished the mental health practitioner community and others working with suffering and violence in institutional settings with an innovative approach to engagement in an optimistic and assessment-driven way. Understanding the Interpersonal Dynamic (ID) consultation is central to the book and, moreover, the very application to a broad range of significant psychopathology is highlighted by the careful and considered use of appropriate case material. Not only do the authors present a conceptualisation of treatment intervention based on a comprehensive and systematic assessment architecture, but their account also emphasises, in stark contrast to more traditional psychotherapeutic practice, the notion of inclusivity and accessibility.

I shall look forward to seeing how the ID approach may be utilised for patients with highly resistive psychiatric presentations through the future evolution of the underlying philosophy of care enshrined within this volume, for example, how the approach might be applied to conditions such as morbid jealousy, folie a deux, and extreme obsessive-compulsive disorder. The fact that the book provides a template for engagement with such severe psychiatric phenomena as schizophrenia and paraphilia instils a promising vision of applicability to the full spectrum of psychopathology, which represents the endpoint of the complex emotional world that we all inhabit.

Finally, John Gordon and Gabriel Kirtchuk—and of course their highly esteemed chapter contributors—have produced a "breakthrough" volume with the potential to become a seminal work of importance within this sphere of mental health practice and must be congratulated on their excellent achievement.

APPENDIX I

The ID worksheet and cluster list

Interpersonal Dynamics worksheet

Identifying information
Patient
Name: ID: Date of birth: Ethnicity: Date of admission:
Referral
Date of referral: Referral source: What are the perceived difficulties that the team would like to address in this consultation?: (e.g., is the treatment "stuck" in any way, does the team disagree about the patient, difficulty engaging the patient, does the patient sabotage any progress?)

Further information
Details
Time: Place:
Source of information reviewed
☐ Patient interview ☐ Patient medical records ☐ Staff consultation: Team discussion ☐ Collateral interviews ☐ Other

Summary of relationship history	
Significant others in early childhood:	
Adolescence:	
Adulthood:	
Index offence:	
What was the relationship of the victim to the patient?: (e.g., was the victim known to the patient) Previous offending history? Response generated by health and legal systems? (e.g., sectioned/bailed/no consequence)?	
Current relationships:	(a) with staff
	(b) other patients
	(c) significant others

PERSPECTIVE	EVIDENCE
Time and again the patient experiences staff and others as …	
1.	
2.	
3.	
4.	
Time and again the patient experiences him or herself as …	
1.	
2.	
3.	
4.	
Staff and others time and again experience the patient as …	
1.	
2.	
3.	
4.	
Staff and others time and again experience themselves	
1.	
2.	
3.	
4.	

Brief formulation (according to four perspective menu):

Expanded formulation (including a longer narrative and hypothesis):

Conclusions and recommendations with regard to risk:

Conclusions and recommendations for CPA care plans:

A. The patient repeatedly perceives others so that they are …				CLUSTERS
	D. Others, the staff included, regularly experience themselves as …			
☐	☐	1	Self-sufficiently independent	Allowing independence
☐	☐	2	Behaving as though he/she knows best	
☐	☐	3	Supporting and agreeing	Affirming
☐	☐	4	Accepting and admiring	
☐	☐	5	Treating him/her as special	Idealising
☐	☐	6	Idealising him/her	
☐	☐	7	Attending to and caring for him/her in every way	Protecting
☐	☐	8	Instructing and patronising him/her	
☐	☐	9	Domineering and imposing on him/her	Controlling
☐	☐	10	Manipulating and exploiting	
☐	☐	11	Accusing him/her	Blaming
☐	☐	12	Putting down and humiliating him/her	
☐	☐	13	Intimidating and attacking him/her	Destroying
☐	☐	14	Rejecting and excluding him/her	
☐	☐	15	Deserting him/her	Abandoning
☐	☐	16	Ignoring him/her	
☐	☐	17	Defying and opposing him/her	Asserting
☐	☐	18	Insisting on their position	
☐	☐	19	Over-revealing and intrusive	Disclosing
☐	☐	20	Pouring out concerns and anxieties	
☐	☐	21	Over involved	Reactive Idealising
☐	☐	22	Over sympathetic	
☐	☐	23	Over-relying on him/her	Depending
☐	☐	24	Draining him/her	
☐	☐	25	Appeasing and complying with him/her	Submitting
☐	☐	26	Giving up in despair	
☐	☐	27	Hurt and touchy	Taking offence
☐	☐	28	Indignant and self-justifying	
☐	☐	29	Showing disgust toward him/her	Recoiling
☐	☐	30	Running away from him/her	
☐	☐	31	Cutting off contact	Isolating
☐	☐	32	Keeping up a barrier	

B. The <u>patient</u> regularly experiences <u>himself/herself</u> as …			
	C. Others, the staff included, regularly perceive the patient as …		
☐	☐	1	Self-sufficiently independent
☐	☐	2	Behaving as though he/she knows best
☐	☐	3	Supporting and agreeing
☐	☐	4	Accepting and admiring
☐	☐	5	Treating him/herself as special
☐	☐	6	Idealising
☐	☐	7	Attending to and caring
☐	☐	8	Instructing and patronising
☐	☐	9	Domineering and imposing
☐	☐	10	Manipulating and exploiting
☐	☐	11	Accusing
☐	☐	12	Putting down and humiliating
☐	☐	13	Intimidating and attacking
☐	☐	14	Rejecting and excluding
☐	☐	15	Deserting
☐	☐	16	Ignoring
☐	☐	17	Defying and opposing
☐	☐	18	Insisting on his/her position
☐	☐	19	Over-revealing and intrusive
☐	☐	20	Pouring out concerns and anxieties
☐	☐	21	Over involved
☐	☐	22	Over sympathetic
☐	☐	23	Over-relying on
☐	☐	24	Draining
☐	☐	25	Appeasing and complying with
☐	☐	26	Giving up in despair
☐	☐	27	Hurt and touchy
☐	☐	28	Indignant and self-justifying
☐	☐	29	Showing disgust
☐	☐	30	Running away
☐	☐	31	Cutting off contact
☐	☐	32	Keeping up a barrier

APPENDIX II

The interpersonal circle (circumplex)

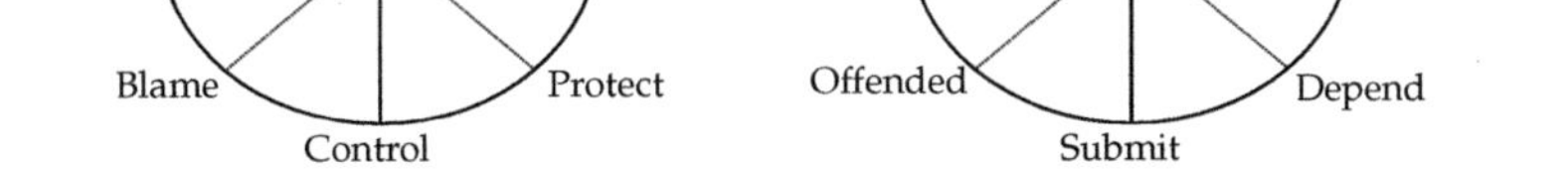

The interpersonal circle: (**A**) active and (**B**) reactive layers, horizontal and vertical axes with intermediate points.

APPENDIX III

Understanding your experience to help your recovery: how to provide ID consultations to individual patients

Beate Schumacher

1. Explain the purpose of the ID consultation to the patient. You could use the formulation suggested under "Introduction" (p. 158).
2. Establish with the patient which clusters from Perspective A resonate most with him by going through the list on pp. 158–159. It would be good if the patient could identify about three or four clusters in all. Some patients may find it helpful to be given the list so they can read through it themselves, others may prefer you to read out each item to them as you go along.
3. The task now is to gather evidence for each of the clusters the patient has identified as applying to himself in Perspective A, and to get a sense of the patient's response (Perspective B) to his experience of others (Perspective A). There is a worksheet for each of the clusters in Perspective A (pp. 160–180) which you might find helpful; choose the three or four which match the patient's clusters.
4. You could use the prompts suggested on the worksheet to encourage the patient to give you examples of situations in which he has perceived others in a particular way. It would be good to elicit about two or three examples, even better if they could come from different periods of the patient's life, for example, one from his current situation, one from childhood, and one from school. The patient might

be put off by you taking contemporaneous notes. If you feel this may be the case, write them down after you have had the conversation with the patient. The most important thing is to facilitate the conversation!

5. When you have some examples for a particular item from Perspective A, try to move the conversation on to how the patient responds to such an experience, that is to Perspective B. Again, you may use the prompt provided on the worksheet to initiate this shift.
6. At the very end (p. 181), there is also an overview list for the clusters in Perspective B. If you think the patient may find this helpful, you could give him a copy of this as you try to elicit the evidence for these.
7. You may wish to have a final run through the overview list for Perspective B to check whether there are ways in which the patient experiences himself which have not come up in response to Perspective A items.

Understanding your experience to help your recovery

Introduction

Sometimes you may feel that your views and experiences have not been taken into account enough. We are not always as good at listening to patients as we should be and would very much like to change that. Understanding how you feel is key to us working together on your recovery.

Perhaps your life has been difficult at times and some of your feelings might be hard to talk about. To make this a little bit easier, we have come up with some common experiences, which we hope will help us to begin a conversation and may help to put your feelings into words.

If any of the statements which follow don't apply to you, just move on to the next one. Altogether, it would be a good start to talk in some more detail about three or four which you feel fit your experience most closely.

Perspective A

1. Have others usually thought of you as someone who can look after himself? Do they treat you as someone who always knows best what to do?

2. Do people usually agree with your point of view and back you up? Do they admire your ideas?
3. Do people treat you as if you are special? Do they think you have something that makes you better than everybody else?
4. Have people generally looked after you well? Do you feel taken care of here, or do you feel the staff are a bit patronising and spend too much time telling you what to do?
5. Do you know lots of people who are very controlling, always interfering with everything? Or people who are trying to manipulate you so they can get what they want?
6. Do you feel that others accuse you, as if everything is always your fault? Do people often put you down and try to embarrass you?
7. Have there been times when you've been scared someone might do something terrible to you? Or have you actually been intimidated, attacked or abused? Have you felt that nobody wants you, nobody likes you, you're always on your own?
8. Everybody leaves you, is that the story of your life? Nobody even notices when you're miserable/frightened/in pain?
9. Are people always challenging and undermining you? Do they just stick to their own position regardless of what you say or do?
10. Are you the one everyone comes to with their problems and worries? Does it feel like you're everyone's shoulder to cry on and that they constantly invade your space?
11. Have there ever been people who've gone out of their way to be nice to you? Do you know what "do-gooders" are? Do you know any?
12. Were you always the one who was expected to sort everything out? Are people often tiring you out by being ever so clingy?
13. Do you usually get your own way? Do most people cave in to you, or just give up eventually?
14. You can't say anything to people, they immediately get all upset and touchy—does that ring a bell? And then they go on and on making excuses for themselves?
15. Does it seem like whenever you come into the room, everyone else leaves, no one talks to you? Do you get the feeling people are put off by you?
16. It's been hard to make friends; people don't let you in, and when they do, it doesn't last. They seem to cut off contact and stop phoning, writing, and visiting. Does that sound familiar?

Worksheets

Cluster 1: Allowing independence

Perspective A

Have others usually thought of you as someone who can look after himself? Do they treat you as someone who always knows best what to do?

It would help me to get a better idea of what it's been like for you, if you could give me some examples. [Please note down examples overleaf]

Perspective B

You said that ... [summarise examples]. How did that make you feel? Perhaps there are some items in the following list which give a flavour of your own feelings:

1. I don't really need people. I am quite independent and generally know what is best for me.
2. I admire lots of people and generally back up what they say and do.
3. I'm very different from everyone else. There isn't anything I'd change about myself. I'm perfect as I am.
4. I am a very caring person, I've always looked after everyone and tried to tell them how to manage.
5. I can be very bossy. I have ways of making people do what I want them to.
6. What's happened to me is my parent's/the school's/the system's/the staff's fault. They've all been useless and I'm never going to let them forget it.
7. I can be very intimidating toward people. If they frustrate or push me, I'll attack them. Or I'll just cut them dead.
8. If anything goes wrong, I just move on. Or I simply ignore people.
9. I don't go along with people. In fact, I go out of my way to do the opposite. I'll tell them in no uncertain terms what my opinion is and make them listen.
10. I've always worn my heart on my sleeve. I really need people to understand exactly how I feel, and I'm not comfortable unless I know everything about them, too.
11. I often get very involved with people. I feel sorry for them. There are a lot who've had it worse than me, and I try to be as understanding as possible.

12. I can't cope on my own and go to pieces when people leave me, so I'm often very clingy. It can be exhausting for them.
13. What's the point in making a stand? It's easier to just do as I'm told, take the path of least resistance. I often feel like giving up.
14. I'm a very sensitive person. I get hurt easily, but I won't let people get away with it. I'll tell them exactly how they've made me feel.
15. I just want to get as far away as possible from everyone. I can't stand them.
16. I'm a very private person. I don't let people in. If they get too close, I cut them off.

[Note down examples overleaf]

Cluster 2: Affirming

Perspective A

Do people usually agree with your point of view and back you up? Do they admire your ideas?

What about some examples? [Note down examples overleaf]

Perspective B

You said that … [summarise examples]. How did that make you feel? Perhaps there are some items in the following list which give a flavour of your own feelings:

1. I don't really need people. I am quite independent and generally know what is best for me.
2. I admire lots of people and generally back up what they say and do.
3. I'm very different from everyone else. There isn't anything I'd change about myself. I'm perfect as I am.
4. I am a very caring person, I've always looked after everyone and tried to tell them how to manage.
5. I can be very bossy. I have ways of making people do what I want them to.
6. What's happened to me is my parent's/the school's/the system's/the staff's fault. They've all been useless and I'm never going to let them forget it.
7. I can be very intimidating toward people. If they frustrate or push me, I'll attack them. Or I'll just cut them dead.
8. If anything goes wrong, I just move on. Or I simply ignore people.

9. I don't go along with people. In fact, I go out of my way to do the opposite. I'll tell them in no uncertain terms what my opinion is and make them listen.
10. I've always worn my heart on my sleeve. I really need people to understand exactly how I feel, and I'm not comfortable unless I know everything about them, too.
11. I often get very involved with people. I feel sorry for them. There are a lot who've had it worse than me, and I try to be as understanding as possible.
12. I can't cope on my own and go to pieces when people leave me, so I'm often very clingy. It can be exhausting for them.
13. What's the point in making a stand? It's easier to just do as I'm told, take the path of least resistance. I often feel like giving up.
14. I'm a very sensitive person. I get hurt easily, but I won't let people get away with it. I'll tell them exactly how they've made me feel.
15. I just want to get as far away as possible from everyone. I can't stand them.
16. I'm a very private person. I don't let people in. If they get too close, I cut them off.

[Note down examples overleaf]

Cluster 3: Idealising

Perspective A

Do people treat you as if you are special? Do they think you have something that makes you better than everybody else?

Would you please help me out with some examples again? [Note down examples overleaf]

Perspective B

You said that … [summarise examples]. How did that make you feel? Perhaps there are some items in the following list which give a flavour of your own feelings:

1. I don't really need people. I am quite independent and generally know what is best for me.
2. I admire lots of people and generally back up what they say and do.
3. I'm very different from everyone else. There isn't anything I'd change about myself. I'm perfect as I am.

4. I am a very caring person, I've always looked after everyone and tried to tell them how to manage.
5. I can be very bossy. I have ways of making people do what I want them to.
6. What's happened to me is my parent's/the school's/the system's/ the staff's fault. They've all been useless and I'm never going to let them forget it.
7. I can be very intimidating toward people. If they frustrate or push me, I'll attack them. Or I'll just cut them dead.
8. If anything goes wrong, I just move on. Or I simply ignore people.
9. I don't go along with people. In fact, I go out of my way to do the opposite. I'll tell them in no uncertain terms what my opinion is and make them listen.
10. I've always worn my heart on my sleeve. I really need people to understand exactly how I feel, and I'm not comfortable unless I know everything about them, too.
11. I often get very involved with people. I feel sorry for them. There are a lot who've had it worse than me, and I try to be as understanding as possible.
12. I can't cope on my own and go to pieces when people leave me, so I'm often very clingy. It can be exhausting for them.
13. What's the point in making a stand? It's easier to just do as I'm told, take the path of least resistance. I often feel like giving up.
14. I'm a very sensitive person. I get hurt easily, but I won't let people get away with it. I'll tell them exactly how they've made me feel.
15. I just want to get as far away as possible from everyone. I can't stand them.
16. I'm a very private person. I don't let people in. If they get too close, I cut them off.

[Please note down examples overleaf]

Cluster 4: Protecting

Perspective A

Have people generally looked after you well? Do you feel taken care of here, or do you feel the staff are a bit patronising and spend too much time telling you what to do?

Any examples? [Note down examples overleaf]

Perspective B

You said that … [summarise examples]. How did that make you feel? Perhaps there are some items in the following list which give a flavour of your own feelings:

1. I don't really need people. I am quite independent and generally know what is best for me.
2. I admire lots of people and generally back up what they say and do.
3. I'm very different from everyone else. There isn't anything I'd change about myself. I'm perfect as I am.
4. I am a very caring person, I've always looked after everyone and tried to tell them how to manage.
5. I can be very bossy. I have ways of making people do what I want them to.
6. What's happened to me is my parent's/the school's/the system's/the staff's fault. They've all been useless and I'm never going to let them forget it.
7. I can be very intimidating toward people. If they frustrate or push me, I'll attack them. Or I'll just cut them dead.
8. If anything goes wrong, I just move on. Or I simply ignore people.
9. I don't go along with people. In fact, I go out of my way to do the opposite. I'll tell them in no uncertain terms what my opinion is and make them listen.
10. I've always worn my heart on my sleeve. I really need people to understand exactly how I feel, and I'm not comfortable unless I know everything about them, too.
11. I often get very involved with people. I feel sorry for them. There are a lot who've had it worse than me, and I try to be as understanding as possible.
12. I can't cope on my own and go to pieces when people leave me, so I'm often very clingy. It can be exhausting for them.
13. What's the point in making a stand? It's easier to just do as I'm told, take the path of least resistance. I often feel like giving up.
14. I'm a very sensitive person. I get hurt easily, but I won't let people get away with it. I'll tell them exactly how they've made me feel.
15. I just want to get as far away as possible from everyone. I can't stand them.
16. I'm a very private person. I don't let people in. If they get too close, I cut them off.

[Please note down examples overleaf]

Cluster 5: Controlling

Perspective A

Do you know lots of people who are very controlling, always interfering with everything? Or people who are trying to manipulate you so they can get what they want?

Any examples? [Please note down examples overleaf]

Perspective B

You said that … [summarise examples]. How did that make you feel? Perhaps there are some items in the following list which give a flavour of your own feelings:

1. I don't really need people. I am quite independent and generally know what is best for me.
2. I admire lots of people and generally back up what they say and do.
3. I'm very different from everyone else. There isn't anything I'd change about myself. I'm perfect as I am.
4. I am a very caring person, I've always looked after everyone and tried to tell them how to manage.
5. I can be very bossy. I have ways of making people do what I want them to.
6. What's happened to me is my parent's/the school's/the system's/the staff's fault. They've all been useless and I'm never going to let them forget it.
7. I can be very intimidating toward people. If they frustrate or push me, I'll attack them. Or I'll just cut them dead.
8. If anything goes wrong, I just move on. Or I simply ignore people.
9. I don't go along with people. In fact, I go out of my way to do the opposite. I'll tell them in no uncertain terms what my opinion is and make them listen.
10. I've always worn my heart on my sleeve. I really need people to understand exactly how I feel, and I'm not comfortable unless I know everything about them, too.
11. I often get very involved with people. I feel sorry for them. There are a lot who've had it worse than me, and I try to be as understanding as possible.
12. I can't cope on my own and go to pieces when people leave me, so I'm often very clingy. It can be exhausting for them.

13. What's the point in making a stand? It's easier to just do as I'm told, take the path of least resistance. I often feel like giving up.
14. I'm a very sensitive person. I get hurt easily, but I won't let people get away with it. I'll tell them exactly how they've made me feel.
15. I just want to get as far away as possible from everyone. I can't stand them.
16. I'm a very private person. I don't let people in. If they get too close, I cut them off.

[Please note down examples overleaf]

Cluster 6: Blaming

Perspective A

Do you feel that others accuse you, as if everything is always your fault? Do people often put you down and try to embarrass you?

That must be awful. It would be really helpful though, if you could give me some examples. [Note down examples overleaf]

Perspective B

You said that … [summarise examples]. How did that make you feel? Perhaps there are some items in the following list which give a flavour of your own feelings:

1. I don't really need people. I am quite independent and generally know what is best for me.
2. I admire lots of people and generally back up what they say and do.
3. I'm very different from everyone else. There isn't anything I'd change about myself. I'm perfect as I am.
4. I am a very caring person, I've always looked after everyone and tried to tell them how to manage.
5. I can be very bossy. I have ways of making people do what I want them to.
6. What's happened to me is my parent's/the school's/the system's/ the staff's fault. They've all been useless and I'm never going to let them forget it.
7. I can be very intimidating toward people. If they frustrate or push me, I'll attack them. Or I'll just cut them dead.
8. If anything goes wrong, I just move on. Or I simply ignore people.

9. I don't go along with people. In fact, I go out of my way to do the opposite. I'll tell them in no uncertain terms what my opinion is and make them listen.
10. I've always worn my heart on my sleeve. I really need people to understand exactly how I feel, and I'm not comfortable unless I know everything about them, too.
11. I often get very involved with people. I feel sorry for them. There are a lot who've had it worse than me, and I try to be as understanding as possible.
12. I can't cope on my own and go to pieces when people leave me, so I'm often very clingy. It can be exhausting for them.
13. What's the point in making a stand? It's easier to just do as I'm told, take the path of least resistance. I often feel like giving up.
14. I'm a very sensitive person. I get hurt easily, but I won't let people get away with it. I'll tell them exactly how they've made me feel.
15. I just want to get as far away as possible from everyone. I can't stand them.
16. I'm a very private person. I don't let people in. If they get too close, I cut them off.

[Please note down examples overleaf]

Cluster 7: Destroying

Perspective A

Have there been times when you've been scared someone might do something terrible to you? Or have you actually been intimidated, attacked or abused? Have you felt that nobody wants you, nobody likes you, you're always on your own?

That must be very difficult to talk about, but it would be very helpful to me if you could say a little about these experiences. [Note down examples overleaf]

Perspective B

You said that … [summarise examples]. How did that make you feel? Perhaps there are some items in the following list which give a flavour of your own feelings:

1. I don't really need people. I am quite independent and generally know what is best for me.

2. I admire lots of people and generally back up what they say and do.
3. I'm very different from everyone else. There isn't anything I'd change about myself. I'm perfect as I am.
4. I am a very caring person, I've always looked after everyone and tried to tell them how to manage.
5. I can be very bossy. I have ways of making people do what I want them to.
6. What's happened to me is my parent's/the school's/the system's/the staff's fault. They've all been useless and I'm never going to let them forget it.
7. I can be very intimidating toward people. If they frustrate or push me, I'll attack them. Or I'll just cut them dead.
8. If anything goes wrong, I just move on. Or I simply ignore people.
9. I don't go along with people. In fact, I go out of my way to do the opposite. I'll tell them in no uncertain terms what my opinion is and make them listen.
10. I've always worn my heart on my sleeve. I really need people to understand exactly how I feel, and I'm not comfortable unless I know everything about them, too.
11. I often get very involved with people. I feel sorry for them. There are a lot who've had it worse than me, and I try to be as understanding as possible.
12. I can't cope on my own and go to pieces when people leave me, so I'm often very clingy. It can be exhausting for them.
13. What's the point in making a stand? It's easier to just do as I'm told, take the path of least resistance. I often feel like giving up.
14. I'm a very sensitive person. I get hurt easily, but I won't let people get away with it. I'll tell them exactly how they've made me feel.
15. I just want to get as far away as possible from everyone. I can't stand them.
16. I'm a very private person. I don't let people in. If they get too close, I cut them off.

[Please note down examples overleaf]

Cluster 8: Abandoning

Perspective A

Everybody leaves you, is that the story of your life? Nobody even notices when you're miserable/frightened/in pain?

That must have been very hard. Can you give me some examples so that I can understand what it was like for you? [Note down examples overleaf]

Perspective B

You said that … [summarise examples]. How did that make you feel? Perhaps there are some items in the following list which give a flavour of your own feelings:

1. I don't really need people. I am quite independent and generally know what is best for me.
2. I admire lots of people and generally back up what they say and do.
3. I'm very different from everyone else. There isn't anything I'd change about myself. I'm perfect as I am.
4. I am a very caring person, I've always looked after everyone and tried to tell them how to manage.
5. I can be very bossy. I have ways of making people do what I want them to.
6. What's happened to me is my parent's/the school's/the system's/the staff's fault. They've all been useless and I'm never going to let them forget it.
7. I can be very intimidating toward people. If they frustrate or push me, I'll attack them. Or I'll just cut them dead.
8. If anything goes wrong, I just move on. Or I simply ignore people.
9. I don't go along with people. In fact, I go out of my way to do the opposite. I'll tell them in no uncertain terms what my opinion is and make them listen.
10. I've always worn my heart on my sleeve. I really need people to understand exactly how I feel, and I'm not comfortable unless I know everything about them, too.
11. I often get very involved with people. I feel sorry for them. There are a lot who've had it worse than me, and I try to be as understanding as possible.
12. I can't cope on my own and go to pieces when people leave me, so I'm often very clingy. It can be exhausting for them.
13. What's the point in making a stand? It's easier to just do as I'm told, take the path of least resistance. I often feel like giving up.
14. I'm a very sensitive person. I get hurt easily, but I won't let people get away with it. I'll tell them exactly how they've made me feel.

15. I just want to get as far away as possible from everyone. I can't stand them.
16. I'm a very private person. I don't let people in. If they get too close, I cut them off.

[Please note down examples overleaf]

Cluster 9: Asserting

Perspective A

Are people always challenging and undermining you? Do they just stick to their own position regardless of what you say or do?

Any examples? [Please note down overleaf]

Perspective B

You said that … [summarise examples]. How did that make you feel? Perhaps there are some items in the following list which give a flavour of your own feelings:

1. I don't really need people. I am quite independent and generally know what is best for me.
2. I admire lots of people and generally back up what they say and do.
3. I'm very different from everyone else. There isn't anything I'd change about myself. I'm perfect as I am.
4. I am a very caring person, I've always looked after everyone and tried to tell them how to manage.
5. I can be very bossy. I have ways of making people do what I want them to.
6. What's happened to me is my parent's/the school's/the system's/the staff's fault. They've all been useless and I'm never going to let them forget it.
7. I can be very intimidating toward people. If they frustrate or push me, I'll attack them. Or I'll just cut them dead.
8. If anything goes wrong, I just move on. Or I simply ignore people.
9. I don't go along with people. In fact, I go out of my way to do the opposite. I'll tell them in no uncertain terms what my opinion is and make them listen.

10. I've always worn my heart on my sleeve. I really need people to understand exactly how I feel, and I'm not comfortable unless I know everything about them, too.
11. I often get very involved with people. I feel sorry for them. There are a lot who've had it worse than me, and I try to be as understanding as possible.
12. I can't cope on my own and go to pieces when people leave me, so I'm often very clingy. It can be exhausting for them.
13. What's the point in making a stand? It's easier to just do as I'm told, take the path of least resistance. I often feel like giving up.
14. I'm a very sensitive person. I get hurt easily, but I won't let people get away with it. I'll tell them exactly how they've made me feel.
15. I just want to get as far away as possible from everyone. I can't stand them.
16. I'm a very private person. I don't let people in. If they get too close, I cut them off.

[Please note down examples overleaf]

Cluster 10: Disclosing

Perspective A

Are you the one everyone comes to with their problems and worries? Does it feel like you're everyone's shoulder to cry on and that they constantly invade your space?

That can be a tough job. Could you tell me about some examples? [Please note down overleaf]

Perspective B

You said that … [summarise examples]. How did that make you feel? Perhaps there are some items in the following list which give a flavour of your own feelings:

1. I don't really need people. I am quite independent and generally know what is best for me.
2. I admire lots of people and generally back up what they say and do.

3. I'm very different from everyone else. There isn't anything I'd change about myself. I'm perfect as I am.
4. I am a very caring person, I've always looked after everyone and tried to tell them how to manage.
5. I can be very bossy. I have ways of making people do what I want them to.
6. What's happened to me is my parent's/the school's/the system's/the staff's fault. They've all been useless and I'm never going to let them forget it.
7. I can be very intimidating toward people. If they frustrate or push me, I'll attack them. Or I'll just cut them dead.
8. If anything goes wrong, I just move on. Or I simply ignore people.
9. I don't go along with people. In fact, I go out of my way to do the opposite. I'll tell them in no uncertain terms what my opinion is and make them listen.
10. I've always worn my heart on my sleeve. I really need people to understand exactly how I feel, and I'm not comfortable unless I know everything about them, too.
11. I often get very involved with people. I feel sorry for them. There are a lot who've had it worse than me, and I try to be as understanding as possible.
12. I can't cope on my own and go to pieces when people leave me, so I'm often very clingy. It can be exhausting for them.
13. What's the point in making a stand? It's easier to just do as I'm told, take the path of least resistance. I often feel like giving up.
14. I'm a very sensitive person. I get hurt easily, but I won't let people get away with it. I'll tell them exactly how they've made me feel.
15. I just want to get as far away as possible from everyone. I can't stand them.
16. I'm a very private person. I don't let people in. If they get too close, I cut them off.

[Please note down examples overleaf]

Cluster 11: Reactive idealising

Perspective A

Have there ever been people who've gone out of their way to be nice to you? Do you know what "do-gooders" are? Do you know any?

Could you help me out again and tell me something about what these people have been like? [Note down examples overleaf]

Perspective B

You said that … [summarise examples]. How did that make you feel? Perhaps there are some items in the following list which give a flavour of your own feelings:

1. I don't really need people. I am quite independent and generally know what is best for me.
2. I admire lots of people and generally back up what they say and do.
3. I'm very different from everyone else. There isn't anything I'd change about myself. I'm perfect as I am.
4. I am a very caring person, I've always looked after everyone and tried to tell them how to manage.
5. I can be very bossy. I have ways of making people do what I want them to.
6. What's happened to me is my parent's/the school's/the system's/ the staff's fault. They've all been useless and I'm never going to let them forget it.
7. I can be very intimidating toward people. If they frustrate or push me, I'll attack them. Or I'll just cut them dead.
8. If anything goes wrong, I just move on. Or I simply ignore people.
9. I don't go along with people. In fact, I go out of my way to do the opposite. I'll tell them in no uncertain terms what my opinion is and make them listen.
10. I've always worn my heart on my sleeve. I really need people to understand exactly how I feel, and I'm not comfortable unless I know everything about them, too.
11. I often get very involved with people. I feel sorry for them. There are a lot who've had it worse than me, and I try to be as understanding as possible.
12. I can't cope on my own and go to pieces when people leave me, so I'm often very clingy. It can be exhausting for them.
13. What's the point in making a stand? It's easier to just do as I'm told, take the path of least resistance. I often feel like giving up.
14. I'm a very sensitive person. I get hurt easily, but I won't let people get away with it. I'll tell them exactly how they've made me feel.

15. I just want to get as far away as possible from everyone. I can't stand them.
16. I'm a very private person. I don't let people in. If they get too close, I cut them off.

[Please note down examples overleaf]

Cluster 12: Depending

Perspective A

Were you always the one who was expected to sort everything out? Are people often tiring you out by being ever so clingy?

Any examples? [Please note down overleaf]

Perspective B

You said that … [summarise examples]. How did that make you feel? Perhaps there are some items in the following list which give a flavour of your own feelings:

1. I don't really need people. I am quite independent and generally know what is best for me.
2. I admire lots of people and generally back up what they say and do.
3. I'm very different from everyone else. There isn't anything I'd change about myself. I'm perfect as I am.
4. I am a very caring person, I've always looked after everyone and tried to tell them how to manage.
5. I can be very bossy. I have ways of making people do what I want them to.
6. What's happened to me is my parent's/the school's/the system's/the staff's fault. They've all been useless and I'm never going to let them forget it.
7. I can be very intimidating toward people. If they frustrate or push me, I'll attack them. Or I'll just cut them dead.
8. If anything goes wrong, I just move on. Or I simply ignore people.
9. I don't go along with people. In fact, I go out of my way to do the opposite. I'll tell them in no uncertain terms what my opinion is and make them listen.

10. I've always worn my heart on my sleeve. I really need people to understand exactly how I feel, and I'm not comfortable unless I know everything about them, too.
11. I often get very involved with people. I feel sorry for them. There are a lot who've had it worse than me, and I try to be as understanding as possible.
12. I can't cope on my own and go to pieces when people leave me, so I'm often very clingy. It can be exhausting for them.
13. What's the point in making a stand? It's easier to just do as I'm told, take the path of least resistance. I often feel like giving up.
14. I'm a very sensitive person. I get hurt easily, but I won't let people get away with it. I'll tell them exactly how they've made me feel.
15. I just want to get as far away as possible from everyone. I can't stand them.
16. I'm a very private person. I don't let people in. If they get too close, I cut them off.

[Please note down examples overleaf]

Cluster 13: Submitting

Perspective A

Do you usually get your own way? Do most people cave in to you, or just give up eventually?

How do you manage that? Could you let me have some examples? [Please note down overleaf]

Perspective B

You said that … [summarise examples]. How did that make you feel? Perhaps there are some items in the following list which give a flavour of your own feelings:

1. I don't really need people. I am quite independent and generally know what is best for me.
2. I admire lots of people and generally back up what they say and do.
3. I'm very different from everyone else. There isn't anything I'd change about myself. I'm perfect as I am.

4. I am a very caring person, I've always looked after everyone and tried to tell them how to manage.
5. I can be very bossy. I have ways of making people do what I want them to.
6. What's happened to me is my parent's/the school's/the system's/ the staff's fault. They've all been useless and I'm never going to let them forget it.
7. I can be very intimidating toward people. If they frustrate or push me, I'll attack them. Or I'll just cut them dead.
8. If anything goes wrong, I just move on. Or I simply ignore people.
9. I don't go along with people. In fact, I go out of my way to do the opposite. I'll tell them in no uncertain terms what my opinion is and make them listen.
10. I've always worn my heart on my sleeve. I really need people to understand exactly how I feel, and I'm not comfortable unless I know everything about them, too.
11. I often get very involved with people. I feel sorry for them. There are a lot who've had it worse than me, and I try to be as understanding as possible.
12. I can't cope on my own and go to pieces when people leave me, so I'm often very clingy. It can be exhausting for them.
13. What's the point in making a stand? It's easier to just do as I'm told, take the path of least resistance. I often feel like giving up.
14. I'm a very sensitive person. I get hurt easily, but I won't let people get away with it. I'll tell them exactly how they've made me feel.
15. I just want to get as far away as possible from everyone. I can't stand them.
16. I'm a very private person. I don't let people in. If they get too close, I cut them off.

[Please note down examples overleaf]

Cluster 14: Taking Offence

Perspective A

You can't say anything to people, they immediately get all upset and touchy—does that ring a bell? And then they go on and on making excuses for themselves?

Any examples? [Please note down overleaf]

Perspective B

You said that … [summarise examples]. How did that make you feel? Perhaps there are some items in the following list which give a flavour of your own feelings:

1. I don't really need people. I am quite independent and generally know what is best for me.
2. I admire lots of people and generally back up what they say and do.
3. I'm very different from everyone else. There isn't anything I'd change about myself. I'm perfect as I am.
4. I am a very caring person, I've always looked after everyone and tried to tell them how to manage.
5. I can be very bossy. I have ways of making people do what I want them to.
6. What's happened to me is my parent's/the school's/the system's/the staff's fault. They've all been useless and I'm never going to let them forget it.
7. I can be very intimidating toward people. If they frustrate or push me, I'll attack them. Or I'll just cut them dead.
8. If anything goes wrong, I just move on. Or I simply ignore people.
9. I don't go along with people. In fact, I go out of my way to do the opposite. I'll tell them in no uncertain terms what my opinion is and make them listen.
10. I've always worn my heart on my sleeve. I really need people to understand exactly how I feel, and I'm not comfortable unless I know everything about them, too.
11. I often get very involved with people. I feel sorry for them. There are a lot who've had it worse than me, and I try to be as understanding as possible.
12. I can't cope on my own and go to pieces when people leave me, so I'm often very clingy. It can be exhausting for them.
13. What's the point in making a stand? It's easier to just do as I'm told, take the path of least resistance. I often feel like giving up.
14. I'm a very sensitive person. I get hurt easily, but I won't let people get away with it. I'll tell them exactly how they've made me feel.
15. I just want to get as far away as possible from everyone. I can't stand them.

16. I'm a very private person. I don't let people in. If they get too close, I cut them off.

[Please note down examples overleaf]

Cluster 15: Recoiling

Perspective A

Does it seem like whenever you come into the room, everyone else leaves, no one talks to you? Do you get the feeling people are put off by you?

That must be very hard. Could you bear to help me out anyway by giving some examples? [Please note down overleaf]

Perspective B

You said that … [summarise examples]. How did that make you feel? Perhaps there are some items in the following list which give a flavour of your own feelings:

1. I don't really need people. I am quite independent and generally know what is best for me.
2. I admire lots of people and generally back up what they say and do.
3. I'm very different from everyone else. There isn't anything I'd change about myself. I'm perfect as I am.
4. I am a very caring person, I've always looked after everyone and tried to tell them how to manage.
5. I can be very bossy. I have ways of making people do what I want them to.
6. What's happened to me is my parent's/the school's/the system's/the staff's fault. They've all been useless and I'm never going to let them forget it.
7. I can be very intimidating toward people. If they frustrate or push me, I'll attack them. Or I'll just cut them dead.
8. If anything goes wrong, I just move on. Or I simply ignore people.
9. I don't go along with people. In fact, I go out of my way to do the opposite. I'll tell them in no uncertain terms what my opinion is and make them listen.

10. I've always worn my heart on my sleeve. I really need people to understand exactly how I feel, and I'm not comfortable unless I know everything about them, too.
11. I often get very involved with people. I feel sorry for them. There are a lot who've had it worse than me, and I try to be as understanding as possible.
12. I can't cope on my own and go to pieces when people leave me, so I'm often very clingy. It can be exhausting for them.
13. What's the point in making a stand? It's easier to just do as I'm told, take the path of least resistance. I often feel like giving up.
14. I'm a very sensitive person. I get hurt easily, but I won't let people get away with it. I'll tell them exactly how they've made me feel.
15. I just want to get as far away as possible from everyone. I can't stand them.
16. I'm a very private person. I don't let people in. If they get too close, I cut them off.

[Please note down examples overleaf]

Cluster 16: Isolating

Perspective A

It's been hard to make friends; people don't let you in, and when they do, it doesn't last. They seem to cut off contact and stop phoning, writing, and visiting. Does that sound familiar?

That must leave you feeling quite lonely. Would you mind telling me what have been the most upsetting losses? [Note down examples overleaf]

Perspective B

You said that … [summarise examples]. How did that make you feel? Perhaps there are some items in the following list which give a flavour of your own feelings:

1. I don't really need people. I am quite independent and generally know what is best for me.
2. I admire lots of people and generally back up what they say and do.

3. I'm very different from everyone else. There isn't anything I'd change about myself. I'm perfect as I am.
4. I am a very caring person, I've always looked after everyone and tried to tell them how to manage.
5. I can be very bossy. I have ways of making people do what I want them to.
6. What's happened to me is my parent's/the school's/the system's/the staff's fault. They've all been useless and I'm never going to let them forget it.
7. I can be very intimidating toward people. If they frustrate or push me, I'll attack them. Or I'll just cut them dead.
8. If anything goes wrong, I just move on. Or I simply ignore people.
9. I don't go along with people. In fact, I go out of my way to do the opposite. I'll tell them in no uncertain terms what my opinion is and make them listen.
10. I've always worn my heart on my sleeve. I really need people to understand exactly how I feel, and I'm not comfortable unless I know everything about them, too.
11. I often get very involved with people. I feel sorry for them. There are a lot who've had it worse than me, and I try to be as understanding as possible.
12. I can't cope on my own and go to pieces when people leave me, so I'm often very clingy. It can be exhausting for them.
13. What's the point in making a stand? It's easier to just do as I'm told, take the path of least resistance. I often feel like giving up.
14. I'm a very sensitive person. I get hurt easily, but I won't let people get away with it. I'll tell them exactly how they've made me feel.
15. I just want to get as far away as possible from everyone. I can't stand them.
16. I'm a very private person. I don't let people in. If they get too close, I cut them off.

[Please note down examples overleaf]

Perspective B—Overview

And what does that (Perspective A cluster) make you feel like? Do any of the following statements give a flavour of how you see yourself?

1. I am quite independent and generally know what to do.
2. I usually go along with what people say; they're often right.
3. I'm better than them, I think, better than that. I'm very different to the people I've known.
4. I am a very caring person, I've always looked after everyone.
5. I can be quite bossy. I have ways of making people do what I want them to.
6. What's happened to me is my mother's/father's/the school's/the system's fault. They've all been useless.
7. I can get very angry with people who don't treat me right. If they push me, I attack them. Or I just cut them dead.
8. I just move on. Or I simply ignore people.
9. I can't bear it if people don't listen to me. I'll tell them in no uncertain terms what my opinion is. I'll make them listen.
10. I've always worn my heart on my sleeve. I'm an open book, tell anyone anything.
11. I feel sorry for people. There are a lot who've had it worse than me, and I try to be as understanding as possible to them.
12. I can't cope on my own. I go to pieces when people leave me.
13. What's the point in making a stand? It's easier to just do as I'm told, take the path of least resistance.
14. I'm a very sensitive person. I get hurt easily, but I won't let people get away with it. I'll tell them exactly how they've made me feel.
15. What they did/do, it's absolutely disgusting. It makes me want to get as far away as possible from them all.
16. I'm a very private person. I don't let people in. If they get too close, I cut them off.

INDEX

For Product Safety Concerns and Information please contact our EU representative GPSR@taylorandfrancis.com Taylor & Francis Verlag GmbH, Kaufingerstraße 24, 80331 München, Germany

Batch number: 10725937

Printed by Printforce, the Netherlands